Psychiatry

Editors

arveen Kumar and **Michael Clark**
St Bartholomew's and the Royal London School of
Medicine and Dentistry; Queen Mary and Westfield
College, London

Commissioning Editor: Ellen Green
Project Development Manager: Siân Jarman
Designer: Sarah Russell
Project Manager: Nancy Arnott

Saunders' Pocket Essentials of

Psychiatry

Basant K. Puri
Consultant Psychiatrist and Senior Lecturer, MRI Unit,
MRC Clinical Sciences Centre, Imperial College School
of Medicine, Hammersmith Hospital, London, UK

Honorary Consultant in Imaging, Department of
Radiology, Hammersmith Hospitals NHS Trust,
London, UK

Series editors
Parveen Kumar and **Michael Clark**

SECOND EDITION

W.B. SAUNDERS

Edinburgh · London · New York · Oxford · Philadelphia ·
St Louis · Sydney · Toronto 2000

W.B. SAUNDERS
An imprint of Elsevier Limited

First edition 1995
Second edition 2000
  Reprinted 2003

ISBN 0 7020 2575 5

British Library Cataloguing in Publication Data
A catalogue record for this book is available from the British
Library.

Library of Congress Cataloging in Publication Data
A catalog record for this book is available from the Library of
Congress.

Note
Medical knowledge is constantly changing. As new information becomes
available, changes in treatment, procedures, equipment and the use of
drugs become necessary. The authors and the publishers have, as far as it
is possible, taken care to ensure that the information given in this text is
accurate and up to date. However, readers are strongly advised to confirm
that the information, especially with regard to drug usage, complies with
current legislation and standards of practice.

your source for books,
journals and multimedia
in the health sciences

www.elsevierhealth.com

The
publisher's
policy is to use
paper manufactured
from sustainable forests

Printed in China
C/02

Series Preface

....

Medical students and doctors in training are expected to travel to different hospitals and community health centres as part of their education. Many books are too large to carry on a regular basis but are still necessary for the basic understanding of disease processes. This series of books is designed to provide portable, pocket-sized companions to larger texts such as *Clinical Medicine*. They all contain core material for quick revision, easy reference and practical management. The modern format makes them easy to read providing an indispensable 'pocket essential'.

Parveen Kumar and **Michael Clark**
Series Editors

Preface to First Edition

....

This book has been written primarily with the needs of medical students in mind. It aims to outline the essentials of psychiatry at the level of the final MB examination, and should prove useful both as a book that can be carried by the student during the clinical psychiatric attachment and also as a revision text in the weeks before the examination. The first chapter details the way in which a psychiatric case should be presented. This is followed by a chapter discussing the signs and symptoms of psychiatric disorders, as the student must be able correctly to elicit these. There follow chapters dealing with the most important psychiatric disorders, beginning with those at the top of the diagnostic hierarchy, namely organic disorders, psychoactive substance use disorders and psychotic disorders. Finally, a glossary is provided; this should aid revision.

The classification of disorders used in this book is principally that of the tenth revision of the *International classification of diseases* of the World Health Organization, ICD-10. Occasionally, however, important subjects that are taught and examined at undergraduate level but which do not appear in the ICD-10 classification of mental and behavioural disorders, such as premenstrual syndrome, have also been included.

This book is not meant to be a substitute for clerking patients or attending lectures. Instead, it can supplement these activities. The need to see as many patients as possible with different psychiatric disorders during the clinical attachment cannot be emphasized enough. As Pièrre Janet pointed out, the best textbook of psychiatry is the patient.

Preface to Second Edition

• •

The opportunity of a second edition has been used to update the information in this book and to add some line drawings. In addition, fuller details have been provided in the text of the diagnostic criteria used by both the *Diagnostic and statistical manual of mental disorders*, 4th edition (DSM-IV, American Psychiatric Association) and the tenth revision of the *International classification of diseases* (ICD-10, World Health Organization).

The pace of development of drugs used in psychiatric practice is very rapid, so that the most appropriate drugs to recommend may change frequently. Furthermore, a drug of choice one year might well be withdrawn from general use the following year, owing to newly observed adverse side-effects. Therefore, in general, only the most appropriate class or classes of drugs to be considered for individual disorders are given, rather than the drugs themselves. However, the major drugs in each of these classes, at the time of writing, are detailed in Chapter 16 on 'Treatments'. It is strongly recommended that the reader refer to the most up-to-date formulary available when learning about or prescribing individual drugs.

November 2000   B.K.P.

Contents

Case presentation

As with other branches of clinical medicine, it is important when assessing a patient to be able to take an accurate history and carry out an appropriate examination. The latter, in the case of psychiatry, includes not only a physical examination but also an examination of the patient's mental state. Together, the history and mental state examination allow the doctor to elicit the symptoms and signs of a psychiatric disorder, should one exist. In this chapter the headings under which the various parts of a case presentation should be given are outlined.

PSYCHIATRIC HISTORY

The reason for referral, the complaints and the history of the presenting illness should be given first.

The chronological sequence of each symptom should be determined at interview.

The psychiatric history should ideally be brought together from both the patient and sources of further information (see the section on Investigations later in this chapter).

Reason for referral

Briefly state how and why the patient was referred.

Complaints

These are the patient's complaints given in his or her own words. The length of time each complaint has lasted should also be given.

History of presenting illness

A chronological account should be given of the development of each symptom, together with any precipitating factors. Associated impairments should also be given. For example, for a depressive episode biological and cognitive symptoms of depression (see Chapter 6) should be included. The effects of the patient's condition on social functioning should be noted.

Family history

Give details of parents and siblings, including their:

- Current ages or ages at death
- Occupation(s)
- Health
- Relationship with the patient.

The timing of parental separation and/or divorce, if relevant, should also be stated.

Family psychiatric history

Any positive family psychiatric history should be recorded, including dates and types of treatment received and the diagnoses made, if available. Enquiries should also be made about any suicide attempts.

Personal history
Childhood
This should include details of:

- Date of birth
- Place of birth
- Abnormalities prior to or at birth, and whether the birth was premature
- Early developmental milestones
- Childhood health, including any history of 'nervous problems'
- Any early emotional stresses, including separation (for example because of death) from close relatives such as siblings or parents.

Education

- Age on beginning schooling
- Types of school attended
- Relationship with peers and teachers
- Any history of truancy or other trouble or difficulties at school
- Qualifications achieved
- Age on leaving school
- Higher education.

Occupational history

Summarize the occupational history, giving details of promotion/demotion. Reasons for being sacked repeatedly (e.g. problem drinking) should be explored. Any other difficulties at work should be given.

Psychosexual history

For women, give the age of menarche, any menstrual abnormalities, history of pregnancies and the age of menopause, if relevant. The sexual orientation (heterosexual or homosexual) should also be given. Any history of sexual or physical abuse should be detailed. Sexual and marital history (including any history of infidelity) and any sexual difficulties should be noted.

Children

Details of any children should be given, including any disturbances they suffer from.

Current social situation

Give the patient's current:

- Social situation, including with whom they live with
- Marital status
- Occupation and financial status
- Nature and suitability of accommodation
- Hobbies and social interests.

Past medical history

Give a chronological account of the past medical history, including the nature of physical disorders and injuries, where they were treated, and the types of treatment administered. Any medication, and its side-effects, should also be enquired about, as should any history of hypersensitivity to drugs. Medication taken should include details of any recent immunizations and over-the-counter medicines such as 'herbal remedies'.

Past psychiatric history

Give details of the:

- Nature of the illness(es)
- Duration of the illness(es)
- Hospital(s) and outpatient department(s) attended
- Treatment(s) received
- Any current psychotropic medication being taken, and any side-effects from this.

Psychoactive substance use

Alcohol

Details should be obtained about the amount of alcohol the patient is currently drinking and the amount drunk in the past, including a history of any withdrawal symptoms (see Chapter 4) being suffered from, either at present or in the past. The CAGE Questionnaire (see Chapter 4) should be routinely administered to patients to screen for alcohol problems; positive answers to two or more of the following four CAGE questions are indicative of problem drinking:

C Have you ever felt you should **C**ut down on your drinking?
A Have people **A**nnoyed you by criticizing your drinking?
G Have you ever felt **G**uilty about your drinking?
E Have you ever had a drink first thing in the morning (an **E**ye-opener) to steady your nerves or get rid of a hangover?

Any history of physical illness, injury (e.g. road traffic accidents), legal problems (e.g. driving offences) or employment difficulties (e.g. being late regularly for work resulting in being sacked), as a result of alcohol intake.

Tobacco

If the patient smokes, the type and number of nicotine-containing products smoked and any previous history of smoking.

Illicit drug abuse

Detail the use of illicit drugs both currently and in the past, including the types of drugs, the quantities taken, the methods of administration and the consequences.

Forensic history

Describe details of any history of delinquency and criminal offences, including a history of the punishments received (e.g. fines and custodial sentences).

Premorbid personality

The patient's personality consists of his or her lifelong persistent and enduring characteristics and attitudes, including way of thinking (cognition), feeling (affectivity) and behaving (impulse control and ways of relating to others and handling interpersonal situations). If the patient's personality has changed after the onset of psychiatric disorder, then details of his or her personality prior to the disorder should be obtained from interviewing both the patient and other informants. Summarize the patient's personality prior to the onset of the psychiatric illness under the following headings:

- Attitudes to others in social, family and sexual relationships
- Attitude to self and character
- Moral and religious beliefs and standards
- Predominant mood
- Leisure activities and interests
- Fantasy life – daydreams and nightmares
- Reaction pattern to stress, including defence mechanisms.

MENTAL STATE EXAMINATION

The mental state examination (MSE) is an important part of the psychiatric examination and should be practised repeatedly after carefully observing how trained psychiatrists carry it out. It covers the psychiatric symptomatology ('signs' of illness) exhibited at the time of the interview. In addition to recording information obtained from the interview itself, the mental state examination should also use information obtained by others, such as the observations of nursing staff in the case of an inpatient. This is important because the patient may not always be forthcoming about his or her symptomatology. Thus, for example, a patient who is observed by the nursing staff to be responding to auditory hallucinations may during a formal interview deny experiencing perceptual abnormalities.

The main areas that must be covered during the mental state examination are detailed in this section. Some of these areas need to be expanded according to the diagnosis. For example:

- In depression: expand on **mood**
- In schizophrenia: expand on **mood**, **abnormal beliefs** and **abnormal experiences**
- In obsessive–compulsive disorder: expand on **mood** and **thought abnormalities**
- In dementia: expand on **mood** and **cognitive state**.

Appearance and behaviour

General appearance

The patient's general appearance should be described, with particular reference to any features that may be consistent with a psychiatric disorder (see Chapter 2).

Facial appearance

The facial appearance can also give clues to the diagnosis, particularly with respect to organic disorders such as endocrinopathies (see Chapter 2).

Posture, movements and social behaviour

The patient's posture, movements (including underactivity or overactivity) and social behaviour at interview should be noted. These are often abnormal in psychiatric disorders (see Chapter 2).

Rapport

The level of eye contact and the degree of rapport established should also be recorded. A positive rapport aids the formation of a constructive, therapeutic doctor–patient relationship. A negative rapport may occur, for example, in the case of patients admitted compulsorily against their will, and in some personality disorders (see Chapter 10). The rapport can be indicative of both the transference and the countertransference (see Chapter 2), and should be borne in mind when considering the underlying psychodynamics of the doctor's relationship with the patient, and the latter's response to various types of treatment (such as individual psychotherapy).

Psychodynamic aspects

The psychodynamic aspects of movements should not be overlooked. For example, a married or engaged woman may play with her wedding or engagement ring during the interview because she has anxieties about her relationship; if she takes the ring off completely this may be indicative of an unconscious desire to end the relationship with her partner.

Speech

Note the following aspects of the patientís speech:

- Rate
- Quantity
- Articulation
- Form.

The **form**, that is, the way the patient speaks, is noted; the content is considered under 'thought content' below. If a disorder in the form of speech (including the presence of any neologisms: see Chapter 2) is suspected or found it is useful to record a sample of the patient's speech that shows this.

Mood

Objective assessment

An objective assessment should be made of the quality of the patient's mood based on:

- History (including biological symptoms – see Chapter 6)
- Appearance
- Behaviour
- Posture.

Subjective assessment

A subjective assessment of the quality of the mood as described by the patient can be obtained by asking a question such as:

- 'How do you feel in yourself?'
- 'How do you feel in your spirits?'

Affect and anxiety

The patient's affect (see Chapter 2) should also be noted, as should the presence of any signs of anxiety.

Thought content

Preoccupations

Any morbid thoughts, preoccupations and worries the patient has are noted. Suitable screening questions include:

- 'What are your main worries and preoccupations?'
- 'Do these [worries/preoccupations] interfere with your concentration and activities, such as sleep?'

Obsessions and phobias

The presence of any obsessions or phobias (see Chapter 2) should be elicited. To check for the occurrence of obsessions, the patient may be asked:

- 'Do you keep having certain thoughts that don't make sense, in spite of trying to avoid them?'

It should be borne in mind that obsessions may be accompanied by compulsions (compulsive rituals; see Chapter 2).

Suicidal and homicidal thoughts

Suicidal thoughts should be recorded. A screening question can be used to detect any such thoughts; for example:

- 'Have you ever felt that life was not worth living?'
- 'Have you ever tried to harm yourself?'

If the answer is positive, then this area of psychopathology should be probed further. More details about the assessment of suicide are given in Chapter 14. It should be borne in mind that it is not only depressed patients who may have suicidal thoughts: they are also more common in schizophrenia, for example. Such thoughts may be accompanied by homicidal thoughts, which should therefore also be enquired after. (For example, an elderly man may feel that if life is not worth living for him, then it is also not worth living for his wife. Similarly, a mother may feel that if life is not worth living for her, then it is also not worth living for her children.) A suitable screening question is:

- 'Have you ever felt the wish to harm others?'

Abnormal beliefs and interpretation of events

Details of abnormal beliefs and interpretation of events should be recorded, including their:

- Content
- Onset
- Degree of intensity
- Rigidity.

Abnormal beliefs and interpretation of events may relate to the:

- Environment (e.g. persecutory delusions, delusions of reference and ideas of reference)
- Patient's body (e.g. hypochondriacal and nihilistic delusions)
- Self (e.g. passivity phenomena and delusions of poverty).

Further details are given in Chapter 2.

Abnormal experiences

Abnormal experiences may also relate to the:

- Environment (e.g. hallucinations, illusions, derealization and *déjà vu*)
- Patient's body (e.g. alterations in somatic sensations and somatic hallucinations)
- Self (e.g. depersonalization).

Further details are given in Chapter 2.

Cognitive state

Note that the assessment of memory includes assessing its important components: immediate recall, registration, short-term memory, memory for recent events and long-term memory. If there is any reason to suspect cognitive dysfunction, for example in suspected dementia, it is important to carry out a thorough examination of the patient's cognitive state.

Orientation

If disorientation is suspected, assessments should be carried out of the patient's orientation in:

- Time
- Place
- Person.

Asking the patient to give the time, the date, and the place where he or she currently is, and questions about his or her name and identity can assess these. If the patient is too disoriented in time to give the time or date, progressively less specific questions can be asked until the level of disorientation has been determined (e.g. ask the patient to give the month or season or year).

Attention and concentration

Attention and concentration can be checked by asking the patient to carry out the serial sevens test, in which they are asked to subtract seven from 100, and repeatedly to subtract seven from the remainder as fast as possible, giving the answer at each stage. The time taken to reach a remainder less than seven is noted. The correct answers are:

$$93, 86, 79, 72, 65, ...$$

If this proves too difficult, perhaps because of poor arithmetical skills, a similar test using three instead of seven (serial threes) can be given. If this also proves too difficult, the patient can be asked to recite the names of the days of the week or months of the year backwards:

- Saturday, Friday, Thursday, Wednesday, Tuesday, Monday, Sunday
- December, November, October, September, August, July, June, May, April, March, February, January.

Because concentration is sustained attention, the serial sevens can be administered first; if this is coped with adequately by the patient, there is no need to check their attention separately.

Immediate recall
Asking the patient to repeat immediately a sequence of digits can assess this aspect of memory. A normal person can immediately recall between five and nine digits, with a mean of seven.

Registration
This aspect of memory can be assessed by giving the patient a name and address and asking him or her to repeat them to you. Record whether the patient makes any mistakes when carrying out this task.

Short-term memory
Asking the patient to repeat the name and address given in the previous test, but 5 minutes later, is a test of short-term memory. Any mistakes should be recorded.

Memory for recent events
Asking the patient to recall important news items from the previous 2 days can assess their memory for recent events.

Long-term memory
Asking the patient to recall his or her date and place of birth assesses long-term memory more formally.

General knowledge
The patient's general knowledge can be assessed by asking him or her to name one or more of the following:

- The President of the United States
- The colours of the national flag
- Five capital cities in a given continent
- Five state capitals.

Intelligence
Whether the patient's intelligence lies within the normal range, clinically, can be judged from:

- Answers to the general knowledge questions
- Responses to questions about the history

- Responses to questions regarding the mental state examination thus far
- Level of education achieved (from the history).

Insight

Does the patient recognize that he or she is ill and, if so, that the illness is psychiatric in nature? If the answers to these questions are in the affirmative, does the patient accept the need for psychiatric treatment? The degree of insight is indicated by the answers to these questions. Note that it is not sufficient merely to record that insight is present or absent; for example, one might note that 'Mr Y had full insight into his illness in that he recognized that he was ill and that the illness was psychiatric in nature, and he accepted the need for psychiatric treatment'.

PHYSICAL EXAMINATION

A full physical examination should be carried out routinely at the time of admission to a psychiatric inpatient bed. Candidates for clinical examinations often do not have sufficient time when assessing a psychiatric case to carry out a full physical examination. In such cases it is usually possible to check the patient's blood pressure, fundi, neck (for a goitre), and so on. For example, the patient's pulse may be irregularly irregular because of atrial fibrillation resulting from hyperthyroidism. A physical examination may allow organic causes of psychiatric symptomatology to be found.

If an organic cerebral disorder is suspected a full neurological examination is needed, including tests of the following:

- Level of consciousness
- Language ability
- Handedness
- Memory
- Apraxia
- Agnosia
- Number functions
- Right–left disorientation
- Verbal fluency.

Level of consciousness

The level of consciousness can vary, as shown in Figure 1.1. The neurological terms somnolence (abnormal drowsiness), stupor and coma are described here.

Drowsiness or somnolence

A patient who is drowsy or somnolent can be awoken by mild stimuli and will be able to speak comprehensibly, albeit for perhaps only a little while before falling asleep again.

Stupor

A stuporous patient responds to pain and loud sounds. Brief monosyllabic utterances may occur. Some spontaneous motor activity takes place. (Note that the term stupor is used here in a neurological sense. As mentioned in Chapter 2, in psychiatry the term stupor is used in a different sense.)

Semicoma

A semicomatose patient withdraws from the source of pain but there is no spontaneous motor activity.

Deep coma

In deep coma no response can be elicited. There is no response to deep pain, nor is there any spontaneous movement. The following are usually absent:

- Tendon reflexes
- Pupillary reflexes
- Corneal reflexes.

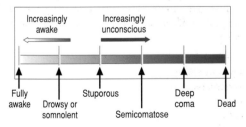

Figure 1.1
The spectrum of conscious level. (Reproduced with permission from Puri BK, Laking PJ, Treasaden IH 1996 Textbook of psychiatry. Edinburgh: Churchill Livingstone.)

Language ability

Motor aspects of speech

Dysarthria, in which there is difficulty in the articulation of speech, can be tested by asking the patient to repeat a phrase such as:

- 'West Register Street'
- 'The Leith police dismisseth us'.

Also check for paraphasias (in which words are almost but not precisely correct), neologisms (see Chapter 2) and telegraphic speech (in which sentences are abridged, with words being missed out). In jargon aphasia the patient utters incoherent, meaningless neologistic speech. Expressive or motor aphasia, also known as Broca's non-fluent aphasia, refers to difficulty in expressing thoughts in words while understanding remains, and can be tested by asking the patient to:

- Talk about his or her hobbies
- Write to dictation
- Write a passage spontaneously.

Intermediate aphasia

In central or syntactical aphasia there is difficulty arranging words in their proper sequence. In nominal aphasia there is difficulty in naming objects. This can be tested by carrying out a word-finding task, such as asking the patient to name objects pointed to, such as the nib of a pen or a shoelace, and to name colours pointed to.

Receptive (sensory) aphasia

Receptive or sensory aphasia, also known as Wernicke's fluent aphasia, refers to difficulty in comprehending word meanings, and includes the following types:

- *Agnosic alexia* – words can be seen but not read
- *Pure word deafness* – words that are heard cannot be comprehended
- *Visual asymbolia* – the patient can transcribe but has difficulty in reading.

Receptive or sensory aphasia can be tested for by asking the patient to:

- Read a passage
- Explain the passage
- Respond to commands.

Global aphasia

This refers to the situation in which both receptive and expressive aphasias are present at the same time.

Handedness

If dysfunction in language ability is found, the handedness of the patient should be determined. The cerebral hemisphere associated with the expression of language is known as the dominant hemisphere. In almost all right-handed people the left hemisphere is dominant. In left-handers the left hemisphere is dominant in about 60%, the rest having either a dominant right hemisphere or a bilateral representation of language functions. In determining handedness it is not sufficient simply to ask which hand is used predominantly in writing: some left-handers may have been forced to learn to write with the right hand during childhood, for example. It is more accurate to ask questions from the Annett Handedness Questionnaire – the patient is asked which hand is used:

- To write a letter legibly
- To throw a ball to hit a target
- To hold a racket in tennis, squash or badminton
- To hold a match while striking it
- To cut with scissors
- To guide a thread through the eye of a needle (or guide a needle on to a thread)
- At the top of a broom while sweeping
- At the top of a shovel when moving sand
- To deal playing cards
- To hammer a nail into wood
- To hold a toothbrush while cleaning their teeth
- To unscrew the lid of a jar.

As part of the Handedness Questionnaire, the patient is also asked:

- 'With which eye would you look through a telescope?'
- 'Which foot would you use to kick a ball?'

Memory

In addition to the tests of verbal memory (a dominant-hemisphere function) carried out routinely in the mental state examination (see above), tests of non-verbal memory (non-dominant hemisphere functions) should also be performed. A given design, such as that in Figure 1.2, should be drawn and the patient asked to redraw this immediately (registration and immediate recall) and then again after 5 minutes (short-term non-verbal memory).

Apraxia

Apraxia is an inability to perform purposive volitional acts, which does not result from paresis, incoordination, sensory loss or involuntary movements.

Constructional apraxia

Constructional apraxia is closely associated with visuospatial agnosia, with some authorities treating the two as being essentially the same. They are tested by asking the patient to construct a star or some other figure (such as a house) out of matchsticks, or else to draw them. The patient can also be asked to copy, at once and from immediate recall, a set of line drawings of progressive difficulty, as shown in Figure 1.3.

Dressing apraxia

Tested by asking the patient to put on items of clothing.

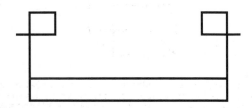

Figure 1.2
A geometric design that may be used to test non-verbal memory.
(Reproduced with permission from Puri BK, Laking PJ, Treasaden IH 1996 Textbook of psychiatry. Edinburgh: Churchill Livingstone.)

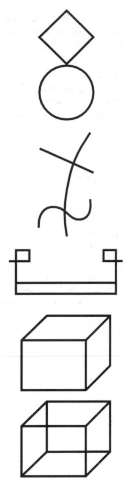

Figure 1.3
A set of figures of progressive intricacy that a patient can be asked to copy, at once and from immediate recall, in order to test for constructional apraxia and visuospatial agnosia. (Reproduced with permission from Puri BK, Laking PJ, Treasaden IH 1996 Textbook of psychiatry. Edinburgh: Churchill Livingstone.)

Ideomotor apraxia

Asking the patient to carry out progressively difficult tasks tests this. For example, the tasks may involve touching parts of the face with specified fingers.

Ideational apraxia

This is tested by asking for a coordinated sequence of actions to be carried out, such as cutting a piece of paper in two using a pair of scissors and then folding one of the resulting pieces and placing it in an envelope. (If there is any evidence of dangerousness from the history and mental state examination, e.g. the presence of homicidal thoughts, then a potentially dangerous weapon such as a pair of scissors should not be made available to the patient.)

Agnosia

The agnosias are considered in Chapter 2.

Visuospatial agnosia

This can be tested for in the same way as for constructional apraxia (see above).

Prosopagnosia

Asking the patient to identify a photograph of a face can test for this. To test for the mirror sign, the patient is asked to identify their own facial reflection in a mirror. In extreme cases the patient may be unable to recognize their own reflection.

Agnosia for colours

This can be tested for by asking the patient to name the colours of various differently coloured cards. The presence of colour sense is established by asking the patient to sort these cards with respect to colour.

Simultanagnosia

This can be tested for by asking the patient to explain the overall meaning of a picture and of its individual details.

Agraphognosia or agraphaesthesia

This can be tested for by asking the patient to identify, with closed eyes, numbers or letters traced on their palm, as shown in Figure 1.4.

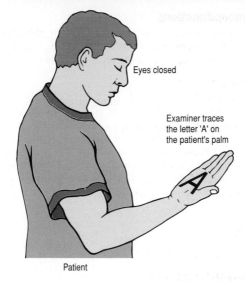

Eyes closed

Examiner traces
the letter 'A' on
the patient's palm

Patient

Figure 1.4
Testing a patient for agraphognosia or agraphaesthesia. (Reproduced with
permission from Puri BK, Laking PJ, Treasaden IH 1996 Textbook of
psychiatry. Edinburgh: Churchill Livingstone.)

Autotopagnosia

This can be tested for by asking the patient to move those
parts of their body mentioned by the examiner, and to point
to those parts both on the self and on the examiner's body.
The patient can also be asked the names of parts of their body.

Astereognosia

This can be tested for by placing an object, such as a coin, in
the hand of the patient, whose eyes are closed, and asking
for it to be identified.

Finger agnosia

This can be tested for by asking the patient to identify, with
their eyes closed, which of their fingers has been touched.

Topographical disorientation

Using a locomotor map-reading task in which the patient is
asked to trace out a given route by foot can test for this.

Number functions

These can be assessed by asking the patient to:

- Read aloud or write down numbers greater than 100
- Count objects
- Carry out arithmetical calculations (addition, subtraction, multiplication and division).

Right–left disorientation

This can be tested for by asking the patient to move his or her right and/or left hands, arms and feet, and by asking for various objects on the patient's right and left sides to be pointed to. The patient can be asked to carry out a command, such as:

- 'Of the two pens in front of you, pick up the one on your right with your left hand and put it in my left hand.'

Verbal fluency

This can be tested by asking the patient to recall, as quickly as possible, as many words as they can that begin with the letter F, in 2 minutes. The number of words is recorded, and the test can be repeated using different letters. In another test the patient is similarly asked to name as many animals with four legs as they can in 1 minute.

••

INVESTIGATIONS
First-line investigations
Further information

On admission further information regarding a psychiatric patient should be obtained from informants, including:

- Relatives
- The patient's GP (family doctor)
- Other professionals involved in the case, such as social workers, community psychiatric nurses, psychologists and hostel nursing staff.

Other important sources of further information include past psychiatric case notes and medical case notes.

Blood tests

Haematological, biochemical, endocrine and serological blood tests that should be carried out include:

- Full blood count, e.g. for anaemia and infections
- Urea and electrolytes, e.g. for renal function
- Thyroid function tests, e.g. for hypothyroidism
- Liver function tests, e.g. for encephalopathy
- Vitamin B_{12} and folate levels, e.g. for dementia and vitamin B_{12} deficiency
- Syphilis serology, e.g. for general paralysis of the insane.

Urine tests

A urinary drug screen should be carried out to check for covert psychoactive substance abuse.

Second-line investigations

The history, MSE and physical examination indicate these.

Further blood tests

Further blood tests that are indicated may include:

- HIV serology
- Assessment of endocrine function.

Further urine tests

Further urine tests that are indicated may include:

- Porphobilinogen
- δ-Aminolaevulinic acid.

Electroencephalography

Epilepsy can lead to psychiatric symptomatology. For example, complex partial seizures of the temporal lobe (temporal lobe epilepsy or temporolimbic epilepsy) can cause the symptomatology of schizophrenia and mood disorders. Therefore, in first-episode admissions of such patients electroencephalography should be carried out, as well as in other patients in whom epilepsy is suspected. In patients with learning disability (mental retardation) epilepsy is common, and this investigation may be required at the time of changing or stopping antiepileptic medication.

Psychological tests

(Neuro)psychological testing by a clinical psychologist can be helpful in many cases, such as:

- Assessment of suspected dementia or pseudodementia
- Assessment of dyslexia
- Assessment of childhood disorders such as attention-deficit hyperactivity disorder (ADHD)
- Assessment of people with learning disability
- Assessment of psychological impairment associated with schizophrenia
- Testing for brain damage
- Assessing specific functions
- Rehabilitation.

Neuroimaging

Structural neuroimaging is a second-line investigation that is useful in cases where an organic cerebral disorder is suspected. Types of structural neuroimaging include:

- Older techniques, e.g. skull X-rays, pneumoencephalography
- X-ray computed tomography (CT)
- Magnetic resonance imaging (MRI).

Although functional neuroimaging techniques, which map cerebral metabolism and regional cerebral blood flow (rCBF), are not routinely used as second-line investigations clinically at the time of writing, their use is increasing (for example in the differential diagnosis of different causes of dementia). Types of functional neuroimaging include:

- Older techniques, e.g. ^{133}Xe single-photon emission computed tomography (^{133}Xe SPECT)
- Single-photon emission (computed) tomography (SPET) with newer radioligands such as ^{99m}Tc-HMPAO
- Positron emission tomography (PET)
- Functional magnetic resonance imaging (fMRI)
- Magnetic resonance spectroscopy (MRS).

Genetic tests

These can be useful in establishing diagnoses (e.g. Down's syndrome, Huntington's disease), and also in presymptomatic testing of relatives (e.g. Huntington's disease).

Sleep laboratory studies

These are used in the investigation of sleep disorders.

....

ASSESSMENT

In giving an oral assessment of a case in a clinical examination involving a psychiatric patient, the following headings should be used:

- History
- Mental state examination
- Physical examination
- Brief summary of the main problems and the relevant positive and negative findings
- Investigations to be performed (or already carried out)
- Diagnosis or differential diagnosis – give the main points in favour of and against each diagnosis
- Aetiological factors
- Management
- Prognostic factors.

Signs and symptoms of psychiatric disorder

In this chapter the symptoms and signs of psychiatric disorders are classified according to the headings of the mental state examination.

DISORDERS OF APPEARANCE AND BEHAVIOUR

General appearance

Self-neglect

Evidence of self-neglect may include:

- A lack of cleanliness in self-care
- Unkempt hair
- Wearing clothes that have not been looked after.

Self-neglect may be consistent with the following psychiatric disorders:

- Dementia
- Psychoactive substance use disorder (of both alcohol and illicit drugs)
- Schizophrenia
- Mood disorder.

Recent weight loss

Evidence of recent weight loss may be provided by poorly fitting clothes that appear too loose. This may result from certain organic disorders, such as carcinoma, and in psychiatric disorders such as depression.

Flamboyant clothing

A patient may be dressed in a colourful flamboyant way if under the influence of certain psychoactive substances, or if suffering from mania.

Russell's sign

The presence of calluses on the dorsum of the hands may be consistent with a diagnosis of bulimia nervosa, the patient using the fingers to stimulate the gag reflex in self-induced vomiting. In such cases the calluses are referred to as Russell's sign.

Hypothyroidism

This may be associated with the following signs, which may be evident from the general appearance (including from the hands on shaking hands with the patient):

- Dry, thin hair (often brittle and unmanageable)
- Facial changes – see below
- Dry skin
- Deafness
- Mild obesity
- Goitre
- Anaemia
- Cold hands.

Hyperthyroidism

This may be associated with the following signs, which may be evident from the general appearance (including from the hands on shaking hands with the patient):

- Exophthalmus and other facial changes (see below)
- Goitre
- Tremor
- Weight loss
- Warm hands
- Palmar erythema.

Primary hypoadrenalism (Addison's disease)

This may be associated with:

- Pigmentation of palmar creases and over joints of the hand
- Pigmentation of recent scars
- Dehydration
- Vitiligo
- General wasting
- Weight loss.

Cushing's syndrome

This may be associated with the following signs that may be evident from the general appearance:

- Thin skin
- Facial signs – see below
- 'Buffalo hump'
- Kyphosis
- Bruising
- Oedema
- Striae (unlikely to be visible prior to physical examination).

Facial appearance

Depression

Depressed patients often have:

- Downcast eyes
- A vertical furrow in the forehead
- Downturning of the corners of the mouth.

Mania

Manic patients may look euphoric and/or irritable.

Anxiety

Anxiety in general may be associated with:

- Raised eyebrows
- Widening of the palpebral fissures
- Mydriasis
- The presence of horizontal furrows in the forehead.

Parkinsonism

Relatively fixed unchanging facies may be caused by parkinsonism, which in turn may result from:

- Parkinsonian side-effects of antidopaminergic antipsychotic treatment (used in the pharmacotherapy of schizophrenia and mania, for example)
- Parkinson's disease.

Anorexia nervosa

Anorexia nervosa may be associated with the presence of fine, downy 'lanugo' hair on the sides of the face (as well as other parts of the body, which may not be visible until a physical examination is carried out, such as the arms and back).

Bulimia nervosa

In bulimia nervosa the face may have a chubby appearance owing to parotid gland enlargement; facial oedema may also occur as a result of purgative abuse.

Hirsutism

Hirsutism in female patients, particularly if accompanied by menstrual disturbances, may result from the following causes:

- Normal hair growth, e.g. in some Mediterranean and south Asian populations
- Polycystic ovary syndrome (the Stein–Leventhal syndrome is a severe form)
- Late-onset congenital adrenal hyperplasia
- Cushing's syndrome
- Virilizing tumours of the ovaries or adrenal glands.

Hypothyroidism

This may be associated with the following signs, which may be evident from the facial (and neck) appearance:

- Dry, thin hair (often brittle and unmanageable)
- Loss of eyebrows
- 'Peaches and cream' complexion
- Dry skin
- Goitre
- Large tongue
- Periorbital oedema
- Anaemia.

Hyperthyroidism

This may be associated with the following signs, which may be evident from the facial (and neck) appearance:

- Exophthalmus
- Goitre
- Lid lag
- Conjunctival oedema
- Ophthalmoplegia.

Primary hypoadrenalism (Addison's disease)

This may be associated with:

- Buccal pigmentation
- Pigmentation of recent scars
- Dehydration
- Vitiligo.

Cushing's syndrome

This may be associated with:

- Moon face
- Acne
- Frontal balding in females
- Hirsutism
- Thin skin
- Bruising.

Posture and movements

Schizophrenia

The following abnormal movements may occur particularly in schizophrenia, and sometimes also in other disorders

- *Ambitendency* – the patient makes a series of tentative incomplete movements when expected to carry out a voluntary action (see Figure 2.1)
- *Echopraxia* – this refers to the automatic imitation by the patient of another person's movements; it occurs even when the patient is asked not to do so
- *Mannerisms* – these are repeated involuntary movements that appear to be goal directed
- *Negativism* – this is a motiveless resistance to commands and to attempts to be moved
- *Posturing* – the patient adopts an inappropriate or bizarre bodily posture continuously for a long time
- *Stereotypies* – repeated regular fixed patterns of movement (or speech) which are not goal directed
- *Waxy flexibility* (also known as *cerea flexibilitas*) – as the examiner moves part of the patient's body there is a feeling of plastic resistance (resembling the bending of a soft wax rod) and that part then remains 'moulded' by the examiner in the new position (see Figure 2.2).

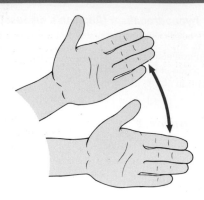

Patient's hands

Figure 2.1
An example of ambitendency. In response to the examiner proffering a handshake the patient repeatedly alternates between extending and withdrawing their hand without ever reaching the point of shaking the examiner's hand. (Reproduced with permission from Puri BK, Laking PJ, Treasaden IH 1996 Textbook of psychiatry. Edinburgh: Churchill Livingstone.)

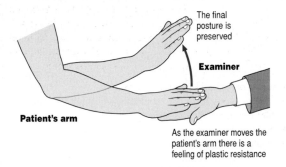

The final posture is preserved

Examiner

Patient's arm

As the examiner moves the patient's arm there is a feeling of plastic resistance

Figure 2.2
Demonstrating waxy flexibility. (Reproduced with permission from Puri BK, Laking PJ, Treasaden IH 1996 Textbook of psychiatry. Edinburgh: Churchill Livingstone.)

Depression

Depressed mood may be associated with poor eye contact, the eyes often being downcast as mentioned above, and hunched shoulders.

Mania
Mania may be associated with increased movements and an inability to sit still. Note that restlessness is also a feature of anxiety and of certain organic disorders (e.g. hyperthyroidism).

Tics
These are repeated irregular movements involving a muscle group. They may be seen in a number of conditions, including Huntington's disease, Gilles de la Tourette's syndrome, and following encephalitis.

Parkinsonism
This is associated with a festinant gait.

Underactivity
Stupor
In psychiatry (as opposed to neurology) the term stupor is used to describe a patient who is mute and immobile (akinetic mutism) but fully conscious. (It is known that the patient is fully conscious because sometimes the eyes, which are often open, may follow objects. Moreover, following the episode of stupor the patient may be able to remember events that took place during it.) The condition is sometimes disturbed by periods of excitement and overactivity. Stupor is seen in the following conditions:

- Catatonic stupor
- Depressive stupor
- Manic stupor
- Epilepsy
- Hysteria.

Depressive retardation
This is a form of psychomotor retardation (slowed movements and thinking) occurring in depression which, in its extreme form, merges with depressive stupor.

Obsessional slowness
This refers to slowed movements that may be secondary to repeated doubts and compulsive rituals.

Overactivity

Psychomotor agitation

There is excess overactivity, which is usually unproductive, and restlessness.

Hyperkinesis

There is overactivity, distractibility, impulsivity and excitability. It is seen particularly in children and adolescents.

Somnambulism

In this condition (also known as sleepwalking) a person who rises from sleep and is not fully aware of the surroundings carries out a complex sequence of behaviours.

Compulsion

This is a repetitive and stereotyped seemingly purposeful behaviour. It is also referred to as a compulsive ritual and is the motor component of an obsessional thought. Examples of compulsions include:

- Checking rituals, in which the patient may repeatedly check that the front door is closed or that electrical switches are in the 'off' position, for example
- Cleaning rituals, in which the patient may repeatedly wash his or her hands, sometimes even to the point that the skin is damaged
- Counting rituals
- Dressing rituals
- Dipsomania: a compulsion to drink alcohol
- Polydipsia: a compulsion to drink water
- Kleptomania: a compulsion to steal
- Trichotillomania: a compulsion to pull out one's hair
- Satyriasis: a compulsive need in the male to engage in sexual intercourse
- Nymphomania: a compulsive need in the female to engage in sexual intercourse.

Social behaviour

Dementia

The patient may not act according to accepted conventions, for example by ignoring the interviewer.

Schizophrenia
The patient may act in a bizarre, aggressive or suspicious manner.

Mania
The patient may flirt with the interviewer and be sexually or otherwise disinhibited.

....

DISORDERS OF SPEECH
Disorders of rate and quantity
Increased rate
The rate of speech may be increased in mania.

Decreased rate
The rate of speech may be decreased in:

- Dementia
- Depression.

Increased quantity
The quantity of speech may be increased in:

- Mania
- Anxiety.

Decreased quantity
The quantity of speech may be decreased in:

- Dementia
- Schizophrenia
- Depression.

Pressure of speech
The speech is increased in both quantity and rate and is difficult to interrupt.

Logorrhoea (volubility)
The speech is fluent and rambling, with the use of many words.

Poverty of speech
The speech is markedly reduced in quantity, with perhaps only occasional monosyllabic replies to questions.

Mutism
Total loss of speech occurs.

Dysarthria
This is difficulty in the articulation of speech.

Dysprosody
This is the loss of the normal melody of speech.

Stammering
Pauses and the repetition of parts of words break the flow of speech.

Disorders of the form of speech

Flight of ideas
The speech consists of a stream of accelerated thoughts with abrupt changes between topics and no central direction. The connections between thoughts may be based on:

- Chance relationships
- Verbal associations, e.g. alliteration and assonance
- Clang associations (using words with a similar sound) and punning (using the same word with more than one meaning)
- Distracting stimuli.

Circumstantiality
Speech indicates slowed thinking incorporating unnecessary trivial details. The goal of thought is finally, but slowly, reached, as shown in Figure 2.3.

Passing by the point (vorbeigehen)
The answers to questions, though obviously wrong, show that the questions have been understood. For example, if asked 'What colour is grass?', the patient may answer 'Blue'. It is seen in the Ganser syndrome, first described in criminals awaiting trial.

Talking past the point (vorbeireden)
The point of what is being said is never quite reached.

Neologism
A word is newly made up, or an everyday word is used in a special way.

Perseveration (of speech and movement)
Mental operations carry on beyond the point at which they are appropriate.

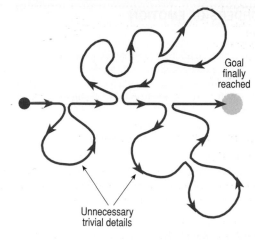

Figure 2.3
Diagrammatic representation of circumstantiality, showing how the goal of the thoughts is finally reached. (Reproduced with permission from Puri BK, Laking PJ, Treasaden IH 1996 Textbook of psychiatry. Edinburgh: Churchill Livingstone.)

- *Palilalia* – a word is repeated with increasing frequency
- *Logoclonia* – the last syllable of the last word is repeated.

Echolalia

Another's speech is automatically imitated.

Thought blocking

A sudden interruption in the train of thought occurs, leaving a 'blank', after which what was being said cannot be recalled.

Disorders (loosening) of association (formal thought disorder)

This is a language disorder seen in schizophrenia. For example:

- *Knight's move thinking* – odd, tangential associations between ideas lead to disruptions in the smooth continuity of speech.
- *Word salad (schizophasia or speech confusion)* – the speech is an incoherent and incomprehensible mix of words and phrases.

DISORDERS OF EMOTION
Affect

Affect is a pattern of observable behaviours that expresses a subjectively experienced feeling state (emotion), and is variable over time in response to changing emotional states (DSM-IV). It may be abnormal by being inappropriate, blunted, flat or labile. For example, if a man appears cheerful immediately following the death of a loved one his affect is inappropriate. A reduction in emotional expression occurs if the affect is blunted. If the affect is flat there is almost no emotional expression at all, and the patient typically has an immobile face and monotonous voice. A person's affect is labile if it repeatedly and rapidly shifts, for example from sadness to anger.

Inappropriate affect
This is an affect which is inappropriate to the thought or speech it accompanies.

Blunted affect
Here the externalized feeling tone is severely reduced.

Flat affect
This consists of a total or almost total absence of signs of expression of affect.

Labile affect
There is a labile externalized feeling tone which is not related to environmental stimuli.

Mood

Mood is a pervasive and sustained emotion which, in the extreme, markedly colours the person's perception of the world (DSM-IV).

Dysphoria
This is an unpleasant mood.

Depression
This is a low or depressed mood that may be accompanied by **anhedonia**, in which the ability to enjoy regular and

pleasurable activities is lost. In normal **grief** or mourning the sadness is appropriate to the loss.

Elevated mood
This is a mood more cheerful than normal. It is not necessarily pathological.

Expansive mood
Feelings are expressed without restraint, and self-importance may be overrated.

Euphoric mood
This is an exaggerated feeling of well-being. It is pathological.

Ecstasy
This is a feeling of intense rapture.

Irritability
A liability to outbursts or a state of reduced control over aggressive impulses towards others. It may be a trait of personality or it may accompany anxiety. It also occurs during the premenstrual syndrome.

Alexithymia
This is difficulty in being aware of or describing one's emotions.

Others
Agitation
This is excessive motor activity with a feeling of inner tension.

Ambivalence
This is the simultaneous presence of opposing impulses towards the same thing.

Anxiety
This is a feeling of apprehension or tension caused by anticipating an external or internal danger, for example:

- *Phobic anxiety* – the focus of anxiety is avoided
- *Free-floating anxiety* – pervasive and unfocused anxiety
- *Panic attacks* – acute, episodic, intense anxiety attacks with or without physiological symptoms.

Fear
This is anxiety caused by a recognized real danger.

Tension
This is an unpleasant increase in psychomotor activity.

Apathy
This is detachment or indifference and a loss of emotional tone and the ability to feel pleasure.

DISORDERS OF THOUGHT CONTENT

These are concerned with the contents of the subject's thoughts, as opposed to how the thoughts are put together (form of thought).

Obsession
Repetitive, senseless thoughts are recognized as being irrational by the patient and, at least initially, are unsuccessfully resisted. Themes include:

- Fear of causing harm
- Dirt and contamination
- Aggression
- Sexual
- Religious, e.g. a religious person may have distressing recurrent blasphemous thoughts.

Phobia
A phobia is a persistent irrational fear of an activity, object or situation, leading to avoidance. The fear is out of proportion to the real danger and cannot be reasoned away, being out of voluntary control. Important groups of phobias include:

- *Simple phobia*, for example a fear of spiders
- *Social phobia* – a fear of personal interactions in a public setting, such as public speaking, eating in public, and meeting people
- *Agoraphobia* – literally a fear of the marketplace, this is a syndrome with a generalized high anxiety level and multiple phobic symptoms; it may include fears of crowds, open and closed spaces, shopping, social situations, and travelling by bus or train.

Hypochondriasis

Hypochondriasis refers to a preoccupation, not based on real organic pathology, with a fear of having a serious physical illness. Physical sensations are unrealistically interpreted as being abnormal.

....

ABNORMAL BELIEFS AND INTERPRETATION OF EVENTS

Overvalued idea

An unreasonable and sustained intense preoccupation maintained with less than delusional intensity is described as an overvalued idea. The belief is demonstrably false and not one normally held by others of the same subculture. There is a marked associated emotional investment.

Delusion

A delusion is a false personal belief based on incorrect inferences about external reality and firmly sustained in spite of what almost everyone else believes, and in spite of what constitutes incontrovertible and obvious proof or evidence to the contrary. The belief is not one normally held by others of the same subculture (DSM-IV). Delusions can be mood congruent or mood incongruent. Passivity phenomena are described below. Some other important types of delusions are shown in Table 2.1.

Primary delusion

A primary delusion arises fully formed without any discernible connection with previous events. It may be preceded by a **delusional mood**, in which there is an awareness of something unusual and threatening occurring.

Passivity phenomena

These are delusional beliefs that an external agency is controlling aspects of the self that are normally entirely under one's own control. Such aspects include:

- Thoughts (**thought alienation**) – the patient believes that his or her thoughts are under the control of an outside agency, or that others are participating in his or her thinking

Table 2.1 Types of delusion

Type of delusion	Delusional belief
Persecutory (querulant delusion)	One is being persecuted
Of poverty	One is in poverty
Of reference	The behaviour of others, and objects and events such as television and radio broadcasts and newspaper reports, refers to oneself in particular; when similar thoughts are held with less than delusional intensity they are called *ideas of reference*
Of self-accusation	One's guilt
Erotomania (de Clérambault's syndrome)	Another person is deeply in love with one (usually occurs in women, with the object often being a man of much higher social status)
Of infidelity (pathological jealousy, delusional jealousy, Othello syndrome)	One's spouse or lover is being unfaithful
Of grandeur	Exaggerated belief of one's own power and importance
Of doubles (*l'illusion de sosies*, seen in Capgras' syndrome)	A person known to the patient has been replaced by a double
Fregoli syndrome	A familiar person has taken on different appearances and is recognized in other people
Nihilistic	Others, oneself or the world do not exist, or are about to cease to exist
Somatic	Delusional belief pertaining to the functioning of one's body
Bizarre	Belief is totally implausible and bizarre
Systematized	A group of delusions united by a single theme, or a delusion with multiple elaborations

- Feelings (**made feelings**) – the patient may feel that his or her own feelings have been removed, and that an external agency is controlling them
- Will (**made impulses**) – the patient may feel that his or her own free will has been removed and that an external agency is controlling his or her impulses

- Actions (**made actions [made acts]**) – the patient may feel that his or her own free will has been removed and that an external agency is controlling his or her actions
- Sensations (**somatic passivity**) – the patient has the feeling that he or she is a passive recipient of somatic or bodily sensations from an external agency.

  Important types of thought alienation include:

- **Thought insertion** – the patient believes that thoughts are being put into his or her mind by an external agency
- **Thought withdrawal** – the patient believes that thoughts are being removed from his or her mind by an external agency
- **Thought broadcasting** – the patient believes that his or her thoughts are being 'read' by others, as if they were being broadcast.

Delusional perception

A new and delusional significance is attached to a familiar real perception without any logical reason.

....

ABNORMAL EXPERIENCES
Sensory distortions
Changes in intensity
Sensations may appear increased (**hyperaesthesia**) or decreased (**hypoaesthesia**). Hyperacusis is an increased sensitivity to sounds.

Changes in quality
In the case of visual stimuli this may cause **visual distortions**. When perceptions are coloured, for example because of toxins or retinal damage, they are named after the colours, such as:

- Chloropsia – green
- Erythropsia – red
- Xanthopsia – yellow.

Changes in spatial form
In **macropsia** objects appear larger or nearer, whereas in **micropsia** they appear smaller or further away.

Sensory deceptions

Illusion

An illusion is a false perception of a real external stimulus.

Hallucination

This is a false sensory perception occurring in the absence of a real external stimulus. It is perceived as being located in objective space and as having the same realistic qualities as normal perceptions. It is not subject to conscious manipulation and indicates a psychotic disturbance only when there is also impaired reality testing. Hallucinations can be mood congruent or mood incongruent. They can be classified as being elementary (e.g. bangs and whistles) or complex (e.g. hearing a voice, musical hallucinations, seeing a face). Modalities in which hallucinations may occur include:

- *Auditory* – these may occur in depression (particularly second-person hallucinations of a derogative nature), in schizophrenia (particularly third-person hallucinations and running commentaries), and as a result of organic disorders (e.g. complex partial seizures of the temporal lobe) and psychoactive substance use (e.g. alcoholic hallucinosis and following the use of amphetamines)
- *Visual* – these are particularly indicative of organic disorders
- *Olfactory*
- *Gustatory*
- *Somatic* – these include:
  - Tactile hallucinations (also known as haptic hallucinations), which are superficial and usually involve sensations on or just under the skin in the absence of a real stimulus; these include the sensation of insects crawling under the skin (called **formication**)
  - Visceral hallucinations of deep sensations.

  Other special types of hallucination include:

- *Hallucinosis* – hallucinations (usually auditory) occur in clear consciousness, usually as a result of chronic alcohol abuse
- *Reflex* – a stimulus in one sensory field leads to a hallucination in another

- *Functional* – the stimulus causing the hallucination is experienced in addition to the hallucination itself
- *Autoscopy* (also called the *phantom mirror image*) – the patient sees himself or herself and knows that it is he or she
- *Extracampine* – the hallucination occurs outside the patient's sensory field
- *Trailing phenomenon* – moving objects are seen as a series of discrete discontinuous images, usually as a result of taking hallucinogens
- *Hypnopompic* – the hallucination (usually visual or auditory) occurs while waking from sleep; it can occur in normal people
- *Hypnagogic* – the hallucination (usually visual or auditory) occurs while falling asleep; it can occur in normal people.

Pseudohallucination

This is a form of imagery arising in the subjective inner space of the mind and lacking the substantiality of normal perceptions. It is not subject to conscious manipulation.

Disorders of self-awareness (ego disorders)

These include **depersonalization**, in which the subject feels altered or not real in some way, and **derealization**, in which the surroundings do not seem real. Both may occur in normal people (for example when tired).

COGNITIVE DISORDERS
Disorders of attention
Distractibility
Here the patient's attention is drawn too frequently to unimportant or irrelevant external stimuli.

Selective inattention
Here the patient blocks out anxiety-provoking stimuli.

Disorders of memory
Amnesia
This is the inability to recall past experiences.

Hypermnesia

In hypermnesia the degree of retention and recall is exaggerated.

Paramnesia

This is a distorted recall leading to falsification of memory. Paramnesias include:

- *Confabulation* – gaps in memory are unconsciously filled with false memories, as occurs in the amnesic (or Korsakov's) syndrome
- *Déjà vu* – the subject feels that the current situation has been seen or experienced before
- *Déjà entendu* – the illusion of auditory recognition
- *Déjà pensé* – the illusion of recognition of a new thought
- *Jamais vu* – the illusion of failure to recognize a familiar situation
- *Retrospective falsification* – false details are added to the recollection of an otherwise real memory.

Disorders of intelligence

Learning disability (mental retardation)

DSM-IV and ICD-10 classify this according to the intelligence quotient (IQ):

- IQ 50–70: mild mental retardation
- IQ 35–49: moderate mental retardation
- IQ 20–34: severe mental retardation
- IQ < 20: profound mental retardation.

Dementia

This refers to a global organic impairment of intellectual functioning without impairment of consciousness (see Chapter 3).

Pseudodementia

This is similar clinically to dementia but has a non-organic cause, for example depression.

Disorders of consciousness

These include, progressively, somnolence, stupor, semicoma and coma, described in Chapter 1; the term stupor is used here in its neurological rather than its psychiatric sense.

Clouding of consciousness
The patient is drowsy and does not react completely to stimuli. There is disturbance of attention, concentration, memory, orientation and thinking.

Delirium
The patient is bewildered, disorientated and restless. There may be associated fear and hallucinations (see Chapter 3).

Fugue
This is a state of wandering from the usual surroundings and loss of memory.

Aphasias

See also Chapter 1.

Receptive (sensory) aphasia
Difficulty is experienced in comprehending word meanings, for example:

- *Agnosic alexia* – words can be seen but not read
- *Pure word deafness* – words that are heard cannot be comprehended
- *Visual asymbolia* – words can be transcribed but not read.

Intermediate aphasia
This includes:

- *Nominal aphasia* – difficulty in naming objects
- *Central (syntactical) aphasia* – difficulty in arranging words in their correct sequence.

Expressive (motor) aphasia
Difficulty is experienced in expressing thoughts in words, but comprehension remains.

Global aphasia
Both receptive and expressive aphasia are present at the same time.

Jargon aphasia
Incoherent, meaningless, neologistic speech.

Agnosias and disorders of body image

Agnosia is an inability to interpret and recognize the significance of sensory information, which does *not* result from:

- Impairment of the sensory pathways
- Mental deterioration
- Disorders of consciousness
- Attention disorder
- (In the case of an object) a lack of familiarity with the object.

Visuospatial agnosia

This is similar to **constructional apraxia** (see Chapter 1).

Visual (object) agnosia

Here a familiar object that can be seen though not recognized by sight, can be recognized through another modality such as touch or hearing.

Prosopagnosia

This is an inability to recognize faces. In extreme cases the patient may be unable to recognize their own reflection in the mirror. For example, in advanced Alzheimer's disease a patient may misidentify their own mirrored reflection, a phenomenon known as the **mirror sign**.

Agnosia for colours

Here the patient is unable correctly to name colours, although colour sense is still present.

Simultanagnosia

Here the patient is unable to recognize the overall meaning of a picture, whereas its individual details are understood.

Agraphognosia or agraphaesthesia

Here the patient is unable correctly to identify, with closed eyes, numbers or letters traced on their palm.

Anosognosia

Here there is a lack of awareness of disease, particularly of hemiplegia (most often following a right parietal lesion).

Coenestopathic state
This term refers to a localized distortion of body awareness.

Autotopagnosia
This is the inability to name, recognize or point on command to parts of the body.

Astereognosia
In this disorder objects connot be recognized by palpation.

Finger agnosia
Here the patient is unable to recognize individual fingers, be they his or her own or those of another person.

Topographical disorientation
Here the patient shows evidence of disorientation on attempting to carry out a task that entails topographical orientation, such as one involving map-reading.

Distorted awareness of size and shape
Here, a limb may be felt to be growing larger.

Hemisomatognosis or hemidepersonalization
Here the patient feels that a limb (which in fact is present) is missing.

Phantom limb
This refers to the continued awareness of the presence of a limb after that limb has been removed.

Reduplication phenomenon
Here the patient feels that part or all of the body has been duplicated.

DYNAMIC PSYCHOPATHOLOGY

Dynamic psychopathology is based on the work of Sigmund Freud and postulates a mental structure made up of the id, the ego and the superego.

Mental apparatus

The mental apparatus is a relatively stable psychological organization within the individual that is involved in both behaviour and subjective experience (such as dreams).

Id

The id is an unconscious part of the mental apparatus which is made up partly of inherited instincts and partly of acquired, but repressed, components.

Ego

The ego is present at the interface of the perceptual and internal demand systems. It controls voluntary thoughts and actions and, at an unconscious level, defence mechanisms.

Superego

The superego is a derivative of the ego that exercises self-judgement and holds ethical and moralistic values.

The unconscious

The unconscious can be studied using the following:

Free association

The articulation, without censorship, of all thoughts that come to mind is encouraged.

Freudian slips (parapraxes)

Unconscious thoughts slip through when censorship is off-guard.

Dreams analysis

Dreams may be based on the subject's unconscious wishes.

Transference and countertransference

Transference

This is the unconscious process whereby emotions and attitudes experienced in childhood are transferred to the therapist.

Countertransference

This describes the therapist's emotions and attitudes to the patient.

Defence mechanisms

These protect consciousness from the affects, ideas and desires of the unconscious.

Denial
The subject acts as if consciously unaware of a wish or reality.

Displacement
Thoughts and feelings about one person or object are transferred on to another.

Introjection and identification
The attitudes and behaviour of another are transposed into the subject, helping the latter cope with separation from that person.

Isolation
Certain thoughts are isolated from others.

Projection
Repressed thoughts and wishes are attributed to other people or objects.

Projective identification
Another person is seen as both possessing and constrained to take on repressed aspects of the subject's self.

Rationalization
An attempt is made to explain in a logically consistent or ethically acceptable way affects, ideas and wishes whose true motive is not consciously perceived.

Reaction formation
A psychological attitude is held that is diametrically opposed to an oppressed wish.

Regression
There is a return to an earlier stage of development.

Repression
Unacceptable affects, ideas and wishes are pushed away so that they remain in the unconscious.

Sublimation
Unconscious wishes are allowed to be satisfied by means of socially acceptable activities.

Undoing (what has been done)
The subject attempts to cause previous thoughts or actions not to have occurred.

Organic psychiatry

Psychiatric symptoms may result from underlying organic disorders, which must therefore be excluded.

DELIRIUM

Delirium is characterized by acute generalized psychological dysfunction that usually fluctuates in degree.

Clinical features

The clinical features of delirium are shown in Figure 3.1. Prodromal symptoms include:

- Perplexity
- Agitation
- Hypersensitivity to light and sound.

Features of delirium itself include the following:

- *Impairment of consciousness*: The level of consciousness fluctuates, often being worse at night.
- *Mood changes*: The patient may be anxious, perplexed, agitated or depressed, with a labile affect.
- *Abnormal perceptions*: Transient illusions and visual, auditory and tactile hallucinations may occur.
- *Cognitive impairment*: Disorientation in time and place, poor concentration, and impaired new learning, registration, retention and recall may all occur. Language disturbance may also occur.
- *Temporal course*: The disturbance develops over a short period (usually hours to days), and tends to fluctuate.

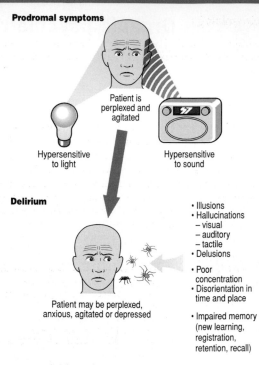

Prodromal symptoms

Patient is perplexed and agitated

Hypersensitive to light

Hypersensitive to sound

Delirium

Patient may be perplexed, anxious, agitated or depressed

- Illusions
- Hallucinations
  - visual
  - auditory
  - tactile
- Delusions

- Poor concentration
- Disorientation in time and place

- Impaired memory (new learning, registration, retention, recall)

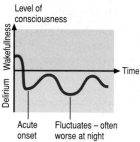

Level of consciousness

Wakefullness

Delirium

Time

Acute onset

Fluctuates – often worse at night

Figure 3.1
The clinical features of delirium. (Reproduced with permission from Puri BK, Laking PJ, Treasaden IH 1996 Textbook of psychiatry. Edinburgh: Churchill Livingstone.)

Epidemiology

Delirium can result from physical illness and is seen in about 10% of inpatients on general medical and surgical wards.

Aetiology

Delirium can result from poisoning, psychoactive substance use withdrawal, intracranial causes, endocrinopathies, metabolic disorders, systemic infections and post-operatively. Details are shown in Table 3.1. This is an appropriate place to consider briefly the more important clinical features of some of these endocrinopathies, particularly those that often present with psychiatric symptoms other than delirium.

Table 3.1 Causes of delirium

Drugs and alcohol	Drug toxicity, industrial poisons, carbon monoxide poisoning, and drug and alcohol withdrawal
Intracranial causes	Encephalitis, meningitis, head injury, subarachnoid haemorrhage, space-occupying lesions, epilepsy and postictal states
Endocrine disorders	Primary hypoadrenalism (Addison's disease), Cushing's syndrome, hyperinsulinism, hypothyroidism, hyperthyroidism, hypopituitarism, hypoparathyroidism and hyperparathyroidism
Metabolic disorders	Hepatic failure, renal failure, respiratory failure, cardiac failure, pancreatic failure, hypoxia, hypoglycaemia, fluid and electrolyte imbalance, carcinoid syndrome, porphyria, and deficiency of thiamine, nicotinic acid, folate and vitamin B_{12}
Systemic infections	
Postoperative states	

Primary hypoadrenalism (Addison's disease)

In this relatively uncommon endocrine disorder there is destruction of adrenal cortex, leading to reduced production of glucocorticoids, mineralocorticoids and sex steroids. The condition often presents with symptoms similar to those that occur in depression, including weakness, tiredness, weight loss, depressed mood and anorexia. The important clinical features are shown in Figure 3.2.

Cushing's syndrome

This describes the clinical state of increased free circulating glucocorticoid and occurs most commonly following the administration of synthetic steroids. Causes include:

- Glucocorticoid administration
- Pituitary-dependent (Cushing's disease)
- Ectopic ACTH-producing tumours
- ACTH administration
- Adrenal adenomas
- Adrenal carcinomas
- Alcohol-induced pseudo-Cushing's syndrome.

Cushing's syndrome may present with symptoms similar to those seen in depression, mania and schizophrenia (including mood changes, delusions, hallucinations and thought disorder). The important clinical features are shown in Figure 3.3.

Hypothyroidism

This is one of the commonest endocrine disorders (particularly in women). Causes include:

- Congenital causes – agenesis; ectopic thyroid remnants
- Atrophic thyroiditis
- Hashimoto's thyroiditis
- Iodine deficiency
- Dyshormonogenesis
- Antithyroid drugs
- Other drugs – lithium; amiodarone; interferon
- Postinfective thyroiditis
- Post surgery
- Post irradiation
- Radioiodine therapy
- Tumour infiltration
- Peripheral resistance to thyroid hormone
- Secondary hypopituitarism.

Symptoms

Weight loss
Anorexia
Malaise
Weakness
Fever
Depression
Impotence/amenorrhoea
Nausea/vomiting
Diarrhoea
Confusion
Syncope from postural
  hypotension
Abdominal pain
Constipation
Myalgia
Joint or back pain

Features of other
  autoimmune disease
  (e.g. vitiligo) are
  quite common

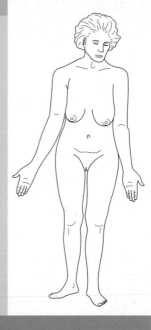

Signs

Buccal pigmentation

Postural hypotension

Pigmentation, especially of new scars
General wasting

Loss of weight
Dehydration

Loss of body hair

(Vitiligo)

Figure 3.2
The clinical features of primary hypoadrenalism (Addison's disease). Bold
type indicates signs of greater discriminant value. (Adapted with permission
from Kumar P, Clark M (eds) 1998 Clinical medicine. Edinburgh: W R
Saunders.)

Symptoms

Weight gain (central)
Change of appearance
Depression
Psychosis
Insomnia
Amenorrhoea/
  oligomenorrhoea
Poor libido
Thin skin/easy bruising
Hair growth/acne
Muscular weakness
Growth arrest in children
Back pain
Polyuria/polydipsia

Old photographs may
  be useful
Symptoms of
  hypopituitarism are rare

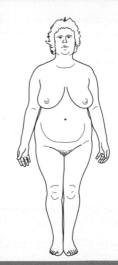

Signs

Depression/psychosis
Acne, hirsuties
Thin Skin
Bruising
Hypertension

Rib fractures

Osteoporosis

Pathological fractures

Poor wound healing

Proximal muscle wasting
Proximal myopathy

Oedema

Frontal balding (female)

Moon face
Plethora
'Buffalo-hump'
Kyphosis

Centripetal obesity
Pigmentation

Striae (purple)

Skin infections
Glycosuria

Figure 3.3
The clinical features of Cushing's syndrome. Bold type indicates signs of
most value in discriminating Cushing's syndrome from simple obesity and
hirsuties. (Adapted with permission from Kumar P, Clark M (eds) 1998
Clinical medicine. Edinburgh: W.B. Saunders.)

Hypothyroidism may present with symptoms similar to those seen in depression, mania and schizophrenia (myxoedema madness). The important clinical features are shown in Figure 3.4. Note that these features may not be seen in children and young women. The former often have slowed growth and perform poorly at school; pubertal development may be arrested.

This condition should be excluded in any young non-pregnant non-postpartum woman presenting with:

- Oligomenorrhoea
- Amenorrhoea
- Menorrhagia
- Infertility
- Hyperprolactinaemia (manifesting, for example, with lactation).

Note also that the clinical features of hypothyroidism may be difficult to recognize in the elderly, as some of them are similar to those that occur with normal ageing.

Hyperthyroidism

This is also one of the commonest endocrine disorders (particularly in women). Causes include:

- Graves' disease
- Toxic solitary adenoma/nodule (Plummer's disease)
- Toxic multinodular goitre
- De Quervain's thyroiditis
- Postpartum thyroiditis
- Thyrotoxicosis factitia
- Exogenous iodine
- Drugs – amiodarone
- Metastatic differentiated thyroid carcinoma
- TSH-secreting tumours
- HCG-secreting tumours
- Ovarian teratoma.

Hyperthyroidism may present with symptoms similar to those seen in mood disorders, panic disorder, generalized anxiety disorder and, in children, attention-deficit hyperactivity disorder (behavioural problems such as hyperactivity). The important clinical features are shown in Figure 3.5. Note that these features may not be seen in

Symptoms

Tiredness/malaise
Weight gain
Anorexia
Cold intolerance
Poor memory
Change in appearance
Depression
Psychosis
Coma
Deafness
Poor libido
Goitre
Puffy eyes
Dry, brittle unmanageable hair
Dry, coarse skin
Arthralgia
Myalgia
Constipation
Menorrhagia or
  oligomenorrhoea in women

A history from a relative is
  often revealing
Symptoms of other autoimmune
  disease may be present

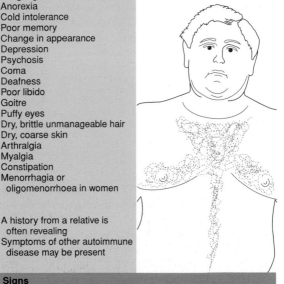

Signs

Mental slowness	Large tongue
Psychosis/dementia	
Ataxia	Periorbital oedema
Poverty of movement	Deep voice
Deafness	(Goitre)
'Peaches and cream' complexion	Dry skin
Dry thin hair	Mild obesity
Loss of eyebrows	
Hypertension	Myotonia
Hypothermia	Muscular hypertrophy
Heart failure	Proximal myopathy
Bradycardia	Slow-relaxing reflexes
Pericardial effusion	
Cold peripheries	Anaemia
Carpal tunnel syndrome	
Oedema	

Figure 3.4
The clinical features of hypothyroidism. Bold type indicates signs of greater
discriminant value. (Adapted with permission from Kumar P, Clark M (eds)
1998 Clinical medicine. Edinburgh: W.B. Saunders.)

Symptoms

Weight loss
Increased appetite
Irritability/behaviour
  change
Restlessness
Malaise
Muscle weakness
Tremor
Choreoathetosis
Breathlessness
Palpitation
Heat intolerance
Vomiting
Diarrhoea
Eye complaints*
Goitre
Oligomenorrhoea
Loss of libido
Gynaecomastia
Onycholysis
Tall stature (in children)
*Only in Graves' disease

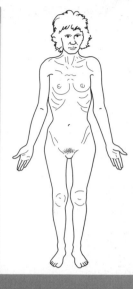

Signs

Irritability   **Exophthalmos**
Psychosis   Lid lag
Hyperkinesis   Conjunctive oedema
Tremor   Ophthalmoplegia
                                Goitre, bruit

Systolic hypertension
Cardiac failure
**Tachycardia or atrial
  fibrillation**
**Warm vasodilated   Weight loss
  peripheries**

Onycholysis   Proximal muscle wasting
Palmar erythema   (shoulder and hips)
                                Proximal myopathy

Thyroid acropathy
Pretibial myxoedema

Figure 3.5
The clinical features of hyperthyroidism. Bold type indicates signs of
greater discriminant value. (Adapted with permission from Kumar P, Clark M
(eds) 1998 Clinical medicine. Edinburgh: W.B. Saunders.)

children, in whom the disorder may instead manifest as excessive growth or behavioural problems.

Management

Carry out relevant investigations. Good, calming nursing care is essential, preferably in a quiet single room. Ensure an adequate fluid and electrolyte balance. Explain the condition to the patient. Encourage correct orientation by allowing the patient to know the time, placing a television in the room and allowing visitors. A low level of lighting should be used at night.

If the patient is very agitated, anxious or frightened, oral or intramuscular haloperidol can be used; if there is hepatic failure benzodiazepines can be given. Benzodiazepines can also be prescribed at night for their hypnotic action.

Prognosis

The prognosis is that of the underlying cause.

···

DEMENTIA

Dementia is characterized by generalized psychological dysfunction of higher cortical functions without impairment of consciousness.

Clinical features
Impairment of higher cortical functions

Registration, storage and retrieval of new information is impaired, with recent memory being affected before remote memory. There is slowed thinking, impaired concentration and impaired judgement, leading to poor insight. Paranoid thoughts and ideas of reference may develop into delusions. Disorientation for time precedes disorientation for place and person. Impairment of comprehension, learning capacity and the ability to calculate also occurs. Language impairment leads to difficulty in word finding, concrete thinking and perseveration.

Impaired emotional control

Anxiety, lability of mood and depression may occur.

Impaired social behaviour
Impaired motivation

Epidemiology

The prevalence of dementia increases with increasing age, from 1% at the age of 60 years to approximately 40% at the age of 85.

Aetiology

The following types of dementia account for 90% of all cases of dementia:

- Alzheimer's disease
- diffuse Lewy body dementia
- frontotemporal dementia
- vascular dementia.

Only brief descriptions are given of these forms of dementia.

Alzheimer's disease

This is the commonest cause of dementia in those over 65 years of age. A 39–43 amino acid fragment of β-amyloid precursor protein (APP), β-amyloid protein (Abeta), accumulates in the brain parenchyma to form the typical lesions associated with this disorder. The numbers of neurofibrillary tangles and neuritic plaques seen histologically correlate with the degree of cognitive impairment. Alzheimer's disease is commoner in women and in those with a family history of:

- Alzheimer's disease
- Down's syndrome
- lymphoma.

It usually presents with memory loss, followed by progressive gradual deterioration. In early onset Alzheimer's disease (beginning before the age of 65 years) there is usually a rapid progression of symptoms, with marked multiple disorders of higher cortical functions; aphasia, agraphia, alexia, and apraxia occur relatively early in the course of the disorder. At the time of writing, there is no intervention that halts or reverses the underlying pathophysiology. Two cholinesterase inhibitors, tacrine and donepezil, are currently approved in the United States, while donepezil and rivastigmine (also a cholinesterase inhibitor) are currently approved in Britain, for use as cognitive enhancers specifically in mild to moderate Alzheimer's disease. Up to half the patients treated with these drugs show a slower rate of cognitive decline.

Lewy body dementia

In recent years the generic term 'dementia with Lewy bodies' was proposed at the first International Workshop on Lewy Body Dementia in 1995. (It was described in 1923 by Friedrich Lewy in a large proportion of his patients with paralysis agitans which had co-incident plaques and neurofibrillary tangles.) It includes various types of dementia such as:

- diffuse Lewy body disease
- senile dementia of Lewy body type
- Lewy body variant of Alzheimer's disease.

It is the second commonest neurodegenerative cause of dementia. Characteristic clinical features include:

- fluctuating cognitive impairment
- spontaneous parkinsonism
- recurrent visual hallucinations
- neuroleptic hypersensitivity.

Antipsychotics should be avoided (or only used with extreme caution) in such patients, owing to a high incidence (approximately 60%) of adverse and life-threatening reactions to these drugs.

Frontotemporal dementia

Frontotemporal dementia is a clinical dementia syndrome characterized by behavioural changes, including character changes such as altered personal and social conduct, arising from frontotemporal involvement and distinct from Alzheimer's disease. Such changes may include:

- disinhibition
- inattention
- stereotypic behaviours

- antisocial acts
- reduced speech.

Mood disorder and psychiatric symptoms of a transient nature may occur and may mark the beginning of cognitive and behavioural deterioration. Spatial skills are preserved. Recognized features of the late stages include:

- apathy
- withdrawal
- akinesia
- mutism
- rigidity
- frontal release signs.

The term covers both the temporal and frontal presentations of this condition. (The frontal variant presents with insidious changes in personality and behaviour, with neuropsychological evidence of disproportionate frontal dysfunction.) Many pedigrees have been described in which the disorder is inherited as an autosomal dominant trait. It is genetically heterogeneous with loci identified on chromosomes 17 and 3. At least three histological entities are recognized:

- Pick's disease
- non-specific frontotemporal degeneration
- frontal lobe abnormalities associated with motor neurone disease.

Pick's disease is commoner in women, with a peak age of onset between 50 and 60 years, knife-blade atrophy of the gyri, and Pick's bodies histologically.

Vascular (multi-infarct) dementia

This ischaemic disorder is caused by multiple cerebral infarcts, with the extent of infarction related to the degree of cognitive impairment. It is associated with chronic hypertension and arteriosclerosis, and is commoner in men. The onset is usually acute and may be associated with a cerebrovascular accident. Stepwise deterioration and focal neurological features may be seen.

Huntington's disease (chorea)

This autosomal dominant disorder is caused by an abnormal gene on the short arm of chromosome 4, containing an abnormal sequence of randomly repeated CAG repeats (leading to the expression of the protein huntingtin). There is marked atrophy of the corpus striatum, particularly the caudate nucleus, and of the cerebral cortex, particularly the frontal lobes. GABA neurons in the corpus striatum are particularly affected. Males and females are equally affected and the average age of onset is 35–44 years. It causes an insidious onset of involuntary choreiform movements which, early on, affect the face, hands and shoulders, or the gait. Progressive dementia follows. Death usually occurs within 15 years of onset.

Creutzfeldt–Jakob disease

Creutzfeldt–Jakob disease (CJD) is a rare progressive dementia that is transmitted by infection with a prion. The cerebral cortex acquires a spongy appearance (status spongiosus). Degeneration also occurs in spinal cord long descending tracts. It has an equal incidence in men and women and a long incubation period of many years. Infection may be transmitted from surgical specimens, postmortem preparations (such as corneal grafts) and from human pituitary glands (used to produce human somatotropin for clinical use). In 1995 in Britain a new variant of CJD (nvCJD) was reported which, it has been suggested, may be linked to transmission, possibly via the food chain, from the neuropathologically related bovine disorder BSE (bovine spongiform encephalopathy). Its clinical features depend on the parts of the brain most affected. The early presentation of nvCJD is commonly neuropsychiatric, followed by ataxia and dementia (with myoclonus or chorea). Electroencephalography shows a characteristic triphasic pattern. Death usually occurs within 2 years.

Normal-pressure (intermittent) hydrocephalus

This is a type of primary hydrocephalus in which the CSF pressure is normal most of the time. It is both obstructive and communicating, and is caused by an obstruction in the subarachnoid space. Peak occurrence is in the seventh and eighth decades. Varying degrees of cognitive impairment and physical slowness occur. Other features include unsteadiness of gait, urinary incontinence and nystagmus. Treatment is usually with ventriculoperitoneal shunting.

CAUSES OF SPECIFIC PSYCHOLOGICAL DYSFUNCTION

Amnesic (Korsakov's) syndrome

This is a syndrome of prominent impairment of recent and remote memory with preservation of immediate recall in the absence of generalized cognitive impairment. Retrograde amnesia (inability to recall events before the onset of the disorder) and anterograde amnesia (poor memory for events taking place after the onset of the disorder) occur.

Aetiology

It can be caused by thiamine deficiency (owing to alcohol abuse, malabsorption, hyperemesis or starvation), intoxication with heavy metals or carbon monoxide, head injury, tumours affecting the third ventricle or hippocampal formation, bilateral hippocampal damage, subarachnoid haemorrhage, infections (HSV or TB meningitis), epilepsy, hypoxia and Alzheimer's disease.

Pathology

One or both of the following are typically affected:

- The hypothalamic–diencephalic system
- The bilateral hippocampal region.

Clinical features

The anterograde amnesia is associated with an impaired ability to learn and disorientation in time. If the underlying pathology improves this can result in a lessening of the extent of the retrograde amnesia. **Confabulation** is a common feature. Other cognitive functions are usually normal, as is perception.

Course and prognosis

These are those of the primary pathology.

Focal cerebral disorder

The localization of major functions in the cerebral cortex is shown in Figure 3.6

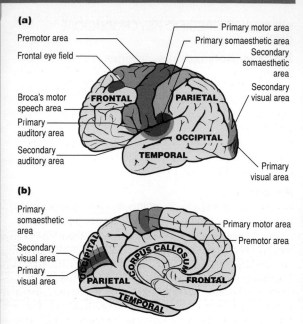

Figure 3.6
Localization of function in the cerebral cortex. (a) Lateral aspect. (b) Medial aspect. (Reproduced with permission from Puri BK, Laking PJ, Treasaden IH 1996 Textbook of psychiatry. Edinburgh: Churchill Livingstone.)

Frontal lobe

Personality changes include disinhibition, reduced social and ethical control, sexual indiscretions, errors of judgement, elevated mood, lack of concern for the feelings of others and irritability. These are related to prefrontal impairment, and in frontal lobe damage are associated with perseveration, utilization behaviour and palilalia. Other characteristic features include impaired attention, concentration and initiative. Aspontaneity, slowed psychomotor activity, motor jacksonian fits and urinary incontinence may also occur. Involvement of the motor cortex or deep projections may cause a contralateral spastic paresis or aphasia. Posterior dominant frontal lobe lesions may cause apraxia of the face and tongue, primary motor aphasia or motor agraphia.

Orbital lesions may cause anosmia and ipsilateral optic atrophy.

Temporal lobe

Sensory aphasia, alexia and agraphia are associated with dominant lobe lesions, whereas non-dominant lesions may cause hemisomatognosia, prosopagnosia, visuospatial difficulties and impaired retention and learning of non-verbal patterned stimuli. Bilateral medial lesions may cause the amnesic syndrome. Other features include psychotic symptoms, epilepsy and a contralateral homonymous upper quadrantic visual field defect.

Parietal lobe

Features include visuospatial difficulties (e.g. constructional apraxia), visuospatial agnosia, topographical disorientation, visual inattention, sensory jacksonian fits and cortical sensory loss (resulting in agraphaesthesia, astereognosis, impaired two-point discrimination and sensory extinction). Dominant lesions may cause agraphia, alexia, motor apraxia, Gerstmann's syndrome (dyscalculia, agraphia, finger agnosia and right–left disorientation), bilateral tactile agnosia and visual agnosia. Non-dominant lesions may cause anosognosia, hemisomatognosia, dressing apraxia and prosopagnosia.

Occipital lobe

A contralateral homonymous hemianopia, scotomata and simultanagnosia may occur.

Bilateral lesions are associated with cortical blindness.

Dominant lesions may cause alexia without agraphia, colour agnosia and visual object agnosia. Visuospatial agnosia, prosopagnosia, metamorphopsia (image distortion) and complex visual hallucinations are commoner with non-dominant lesions.

Corpus callosum

Acute severe intellectual impairment may occur. Left-sided apraxia to verbal commands and astereognosis in the left hand may occur if the left hemisphere is dominant.

Diencephalon and brain stem

Midline lesions are associated with the amnesic syndrome, hypersomnia, akinetic mutism, intellectual impairment, dementia, personality changes and features of raised intracranial pressure.

Pressure on the optic chiasma may lead to visual field defects.

Thalamic lesions may cause hypalgesia to painful stimuli and sensory disorders similar to those seen in the parietal lobe syndrome.

Hypothalamic lesions may cause polydipsia, polyuria, increased body temperature, obesity, amenorrhoea or impotence and an altered rate of sexual development.

Pituitary lesions cause endocrine disorders.

Brainstem lesions may cause cranial nerve palsies and long tract motor and sensory dysfunction.

Other organic mental disorders

Organic hallucinosis

This is a disorder of persistent or recurrent hallucinations, usually visual or auditory, which occur in clear consciousness without any significant intellectual decline (ICD-10). Causes include psychoactive substance use, intoxication, intracranial causes (e.g. tumours, head injury, migraine, infection and epilepsy), sensory deprivation, hypothyroidism and Huntington's disease.

Organic catatonic disorder

Diminished (stupor) or increased (excitement) psychomotor activity occurs associated with catatonic symptoms; the extremes of psychomotor disturbance may alternate (ICD-10). Causes include encephalitis and carbon monoxide poisoning.

Organic delusional or schizophrenia-like disorder

A disorder in which the clinical picture is dominated by persistent or recurrent delusions, with or without hallucinations (ICD-10). Causes include psychoactive substance use, intracranial causes (e.g. tumours and complex partial seizures of the temporal lobe) and Huntington's disease.

Organic mood disorder

Causes include psychoactive substance use, medication (e.g. corticosteroids, L-dopa, clonidine, methyldopa, reserpine, oestrogens and clomiphene), endocrine disorders (e.g. hypothyroidism, hyperthyroidism, Addison's disease, Cushing's syndrome, hypoglycaemia, hyperparathyroidism and hypopituitarism), pernicious anaemia, systemic lupus erythematosus (SLE), neoplasia, infections, Parkinson's disease and head injury.

Organic anxiety disorder
Causes include hyperthyroidism, phaeochromocytoma and hypoglycaemia.

Organic personality disorder
Causes include head injury, cerebral tumours, cerebral abscesses, subarachnoid haemorrhage, neurosyphilis, epilepsy, Huntington's disease, hepatolenticular degeneration (Wilson's disease), medication (e.g. corticosteroids), psychoactive substance use and endocrinopathies.

OTHER NEUROPSYCHIATRIC DISORDERS

These include systemic lupus erythematosus (SLE), cerebral arterial syndromes, cerebrovascular accidents, subarachnoid haemorrhage, neurosyphilis, viral encephalitis, chronic fatigue syndrome (myalgic encephalomyelitis, ME), cerebral abscess, AIDS related complex (ARC), acquired immuno-deficiency syndrome (AIDS), head injury, punch-drunk syndrome (post-traumatic dementia), multiple sclerosis, hepatolenticular degeneration (Wilson's disease), acute porphyrias, Parkinson's disease, cerebral tumours and epilepsy.

Psychoactive substance use disorders

DEFINITIONS

These definitions are based on WHO recommendations and ICD-10.

Acute intoxication

A transient condition following the administration of a psychoactive substance, causing changes in physiological, psychological or behavioural functions and responses.

Dependence syndrome

The use of psychoactive substances has a higher priority than other behaviours that once had higher value. There is a desire, often strong and overpowering, to take the substance(s) on a continuous or periodic basis. Tolerance may or may not be present.

Harmful use

A pattern of psychoactive substance use which is causing damage to physical or mental health.

Physical dependence

An adaptive state in which intense physical disturbance occurs when the administration of a psychoactive substance is suspended. There is a desire to take the substance to avoid the physical symptoms of the withdrawal state.

Psychological dependence

A psychoactive substance produces a feeling of satisfaction and a psychological drive that requires periodic or continuous administration of that substance to produce pleasure or to avoid the psychological discomfort of its absence.

Tolerance

The desired central nervous system effects of a psychoactive substance diminish with repeated use, so that increasing doses are needed to achieve the same effects.

Withdrawal state

Physical and psychological symptoms, which may be complicated by delirium or convulsions, occurring following absolute or relative withdrawal of a psychoactive substance after its repeated use.

··

ALCOHOL PROBLEMS

The concentration of alcohol in beverages may be given as a 'proof'. In the USA $1°$ proof is 0.5% by volume (v/v). In Britain $1°$ proof is 0.5715% by volume. One unit is approximately 8–10 g alcohol (Figure 4.1).

Types of alcohol problems

Excessive consumption

The Royal College of Physicians has defined **low-risk levels** of consumption as up to 21 units of alcohol per week for men, and up to 14 units per week for non-pregnant women. This amount should not be consumed in one go, and alcohol should not be consumed every day, for these levels to apply. Consumption in greater amounts is regarded as excessive and carries a much greater risk of developing alcohol-related disabilities and dependence.

Alcohol-related disabilities

Physical complications of excessive alcohol consumption include gastrointestinal disorders, malnutrition, hepatic damage, pancreatitis, hypertension, arrhythmias, iron-deficiency anaemia, macrocytosis, folate deficiency, nerve and muscle disorders, accidents and trauma, increased risk of infections (e.g. tuberculosis), and increased risk of cancer of the oropharynx, oesophagus, pancreas, liver and lung. Drinking in pregnancy can cause the fetal alcohol syndrome.

Psychiatric complications include depressed mood, suicide, personality changes, short-term amnesia (blackouts), alcoholic hallucinosis (auditory hallucinations in clear consciousness), psychosexual disorders, delusional (pathological) jealousy, fugue states, gambling, the use of other psychoactive substances, the amnesic syndrome, dementia, and withdrawal symptoms such as delirium tremens and withdrawal fits.

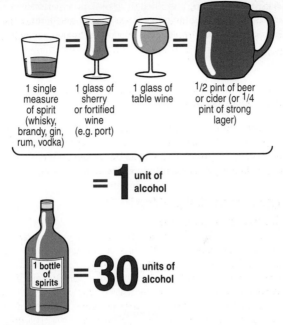

Figure 4.1
Alcoholic beverages and units of alcohol. (Reproduced with permission from Puri BK, Laking PJ, Treasaden IH 1996 Textbook of psychiatry. Edinburgh: Churchill Livingstone.)

Alcohol-induced amnesic syndrome is frequently preceded by **Wernicke's encephalopathy**, caused by thiamine deficiency, which may be reversible in its early stages through abstinence and high-dose thiamine treatment. Its features include:

- Ophthalmoplegia
- Nystagmus
- Ataxia
- Clouding of consciousness
- Peripheral neuropathy.

Social complications include the breakdown of relationships, marriages and families (because of mood changes, personality deterioration, verbal abuse, physical violence, psychosexual disorders, delusional jealousy, and associated gambling and illicit drug use), poor performance at work, crime (e.g. arson, sexual offences and homicide), and accidents and trauma (e.g. road accidents).

Problem drinking

This is said to occur when chronic heavy drinking causes alcohol-related disabilities.

Alcohol dependence

The following symptoms form the **alcohol dependence syndrome**:

- Primacy of drinking over other activities
- Subjective awareness of a compulsion to drink and difficulty in controlling the amount drunk
- A narrowing of the drinking repertoire
- Increased tolerance to alcohol
- Repeated withdrawal symptoms
- Relief or avoidance of withdrawal symptoms by further drinking
- Reinstatement of drinking after abstinence.

Epidemiology

Indices of alcohol consumption

Useful indices are figures for hepatic cirrhosis mortality (see Figure 4.2), drunkenness offences (including drink–driving offences), psychiatric hospital admissions for alcohol abuse, and surveys.

Sex

The prevalence and lifetime expectancy of heavy drinking is higher in men.

Age

In western countries the highest rates of heavy drinking are in adolescence and the early 20s.

Occupation

Occupations at high risk are shown in Figure 4.3.

Aetiology

Individual causes

These include the availability of alcoholic beverages to those in certain occupations, stressful jobs, genetic factors,

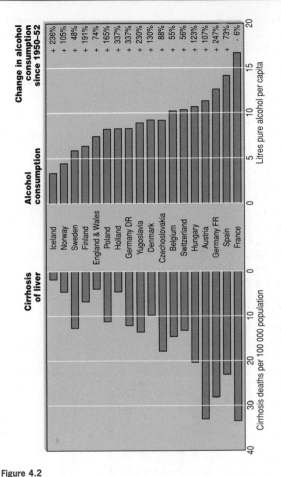

Figure 4.2
The relationship between hepatic cirrhosis mortality and alcohol consumption in selected European countries during the mid 1970s. (After Alcohol, reducing the harm 1981 Office of Health Economics) {Reproduced with permission from Puri BK, Laking PJ, Treasaden IH 1996 Textbook of psychiatry. Edinburgh: Churchill Livingstone.)

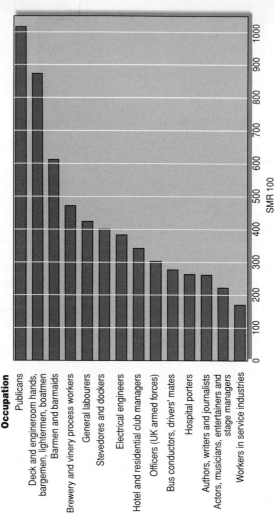

Figure 4.3
Occupations with higher than normal mortality rates (standardized mortality ratio (SMR) > 100) from alcoholic hepatic cirrhosis in the United Kingdom.) Reproduced with permission from Puri BK, Laking PJ, Treasaden IH 1996 Textbook of psychiatry. Edinburgh: Churchill Livingstone.)

personality, advertising pressures, peer-group pressures and the following predisposing psychiatric disorders:

- Depression and bereavement
- Anxiety disorders
- Phobic disorders
- Schizophrenia (e.g. homeless withdrawn patients with affective flattening)
- (Hypo)mania.

Social causes

Cultural factors and economic factors (reduced real price is associated with increased consumption).

Assessment

History

Look in particular for evidence of difficulties at work (e.g. absenteeism and frequent changes of job), a high-risk occupation, psychosexual and relationship difficulties, repeated accidents, withdrawal symptoms, a family history of alcohol problems, and a forensic history (e.g. drink–driving offences).

The alcohol history should include the pattern of drinking and the average number of units consumed weekly.

Screen with the CAGE Questionnaire:

- Have you ever felt you should *Cut down* on your drinking?
- Have people *Annoyed* you by criticizing your drinking?
- Have you ever felt *Guilty* about your drinking?
- Have you ever had a drink first thing in the morning (an *Eye-opener*) to steady your nerves or get rid of a hangover?

Two or more positive answers are indicative of problem drinking.

Mental state examination

Look for evidence of the psychopathology associated with chronic heavy alcohol consumption.

Physical examination

Look for evidence of withdrawal symptoms, liver disease, accidents or fighting, and illicit drug abuse.

Investigations

Further information is required. The following may be raised:

- Mean corpuscular volume (MCV)
- γ-Glutamyltransferase (γ GT)
- Aspartate transaminase (AST)
- Blood alcohol concentration (measured from a blood sample or via expired air)
- Plasma uric acid concentration.

Treatment

If inpatient treatment is needed, sign a contract in which the patient agrees not to drink anything containing alcohol (e.g. beverages, aftershave lotion, perfume) while an inpatient. Aim for total abstinence.

Withdrawal symptoms

Inpatient treatment is preferable, with support and explanation, nursing in a quiet room, rehydration and correction of electrolyte imbalance (if hypoglycaemic, oral or parenteral glucose replacement should be given *slowly, with great care* with *thiamine*, in order not to precipitate Wernicke's encephalopathy in thiamine deficiency), intramuscular B-complex and C vitamins (observe for the rare possibility of an anaphylactic reaction), and a reducing regimen of benzodiazepines (e.g. diazepam or chlordiazepoxide) or chlormethiazole. Note that both benzodiazepines and chlormethiazole have a dependence potential and should therefore not be prescribed if the patient is likely to continue drinking alcohol (particularly in the case of outpatients).

Withdrawal fits

Treat with intravenous or rectal diazepam.

Delirium tremens

The treatment for this is as for delirium in general.

Wernicke's encephalopathy

In its early stages this may respond to abstention and parenteral thiamine.

Alcoholic hallucinosis

Treatment is with phenothiazine antipsychotics, but note that they lower the seizure threshold, thereby increasing the risk of withdrawal fits.

Long-term prevention of problem drinking

A drinking diary can be kept. Psychological treatments include individual, supportive, group and behaviour therapies. Alcoholics Anonymous may be helpful, as may hostels and group homes in rehabilitation.

Prophylactic adjunctive disulfiram treatment can be given. This causes very unpleasant systemic reactions following the ingestion of small amounts of alcohol (even that in toiletries and other oral medicines) because of the accumulation in the body of acetaldehyde; these reactions include:

- Facial flushing
- Throbbing headache
- Palpitations
- Tachycardia
- Nausea
- Vomiting.

In patients taking prophylactic disulfiram, large doses of alcohol can lead to:

- Arrhythmias
- Hypotension
- Collapse.

Acamprosate (taken regularly, usually three times daily), in combination with counselling, may be helpful in maintaining abstinence. This treatment should be initiated as soon as possible after the alcohol withdrawal period (that is, after abstinence has been achieved) and maintained if the patient relapses. Its therapeutic benefit is negated if there is continued alcohol abuse. The recommended treatment period is 1 year.

Prognosis

Good prognostic factors include good insight, strong motivation, and good social and family support. Emotional states, interpersonal conflicts and social pressures can precipitate relapse.

··
OTHER PSYCHOACTIVE SUBSTANCES

A drug screen should be carried out if psychoactive substance use is suspected.

Opioids

Regular use leads to tolerance and both physical and psychological dependence.

Types
These include natural opioids derived from the opium poppy (e.g. morphine and heroin (diamorphine)), synthetic opioids (e.g. methadone and oxycodone), and synthetic compounds with both opioid agonist and antagonist properties (e.g. buprenorphine and pentazocine).

Administration
Heroin is usually taken intravenously.

Actions
The psychological actions of opioids include euphoria, analgesia and lowered libido. Intravenous heroin causes a powerful transient pleasurable 'rush'. Clinical features seen in chronic opioid dependence, include:

- Small pinpoint pupils
- Malaise
- Venepuncture marks sites of infection
- Tremor
- Erectile dysfunction
- Constipation.

Withdrawal symptoms ('cold turkey')
These include an intense craving for the drug, nausea and vomiting, muscle aches and joint pains, lacrimation and rhinorrhoea, dilated pupils, piloerection, sweating, diarrhoea, yawning, body temperature changes, restlessness and insomnia, increased cardiac rate and abdominal pains.

Treatment
Detoxification with chlormethiazole, a benzodiazepine, or, in the case of dependency on heroin, methadone.

Cannabinoids

Cannabinoids do not cause physical dependence but can lead to marked psychological dependence.

Types
Tetrahydrocannabinol is found in derivatives of the cannabis plant (e.g. marijuana and hashish) and synthetic analogues.

Administration
Smoking ('joints') and orally.

Actions
The psychological actions of cannabinoids include euphoria, anxiety, suspiciousness (which may develop into persecutory delusions), a feeling of time being slowed, impaired judgement and social withdrawal. High doses can cause depersonalization, derealization and hallucinations. Some clinical features following cannabinoid administration include:

- Conjunctival infection
- Dry mouth and cough
- Tachycardia
- Increased appetite, particularly for junk food.

Cocaine

Cocaine causes psychological dependence.

Types and administration
Cocaine hydrochloride powder is inhaled nasally or dissolved and injected intravenously; coca leaves are chewed; coca paste is smoked; and crack cocaine can be smoked, releasing vapours. Crack cocaine is an alkaloid form of cocaine that is extracted from cocaine hydrochloride using a reagent such as sodium bicarbonate (baking soda). It is changed into a gaseous state by the application of moderate heat (which destroys cocaine hydrochloride).

Thus crack cocaine can be readily self-administered by heating and inhaling the vapours given off. Furthermore, crack has a rapid onset of potent psychoactive actions, causing rapid and powerful psychological dependence.

Actions
Psychological actions include euphoria, grandiosity, agitation, impaired judgement, and both visual and tactile hallucinations (formication – the 'cocaine bug'). High doses may lead to ideas of reference, increased sexual interest and delusional disorders, as well as physical changes such as tachycardia, dilated pupils, raised blood pressure, sweating, nausea and vomiting.

Withdrawal symptoms
A rebound 'crash' occurs, characterized by dysphoria, a craving for cocaine, anxiety, irritability and fatigue. Sudden cessation following regular use can cause delirium, delusional thoughts and suicidal thoughts.

Amphetamine and related substances

These substances can cause psychological dependence.

Administration
Amphetamines (e.g. dexamphetamine) and related CNS stimulants (e.g. fenfluramine and dexfenfluramine) are taken by illicit users orally or, for a more intense 'rush', intravenously. Methamphetamine ('speed') may also be inhaled nasally.

Actions
Psychological actions include euphoria, a feeling of well-being, increased energy and drive, and a reduced need for sleep. Physical effects include tachycardia, dilated pupils and raised blood pressure. High doses, particularly with chronic use, can cause grandiosity, hypervigilance, agitation, impaired judgement, illusions, hallucinations (tactile (formication), auditory and visual), delusional disorders, and a schizophrenia-like psychosis (which usually subsides after stopping the drug but which may precipitate a schizophrenic illness).

Withdrawal symptoms
Delirium, dysphoric mood (depression, irritability and anxiety), fatigue, insomnia or hypersomnia, and agitation.

Hallucinogens

Psychological dependence may occur.

Types
These include substances related to serotonin (e.g. lysergic acid diethylamine (LSD) and dimethyltryptamine (DMT)), substances related to catecholamines (e.g. mescaline), phencyclidine (PCP) and related arylcyclohexylamines (e.g. ketamine) and 3,4-methylenedioxymethamphetamine (MDMA or 'Ecstasy').

Administration
Orally.

Actions
Psychological actions include hallucinations, intensified perceptions, depersonalization, derealization, illusions, synaesthesia, anxiety, depression (which may lead to suicide), ideas of reference, impaired judgement and delusional disorders (which may be life-threatening). In addition, MDMA causes loving feelings towards others. Physical effects include dilated pupils, tachycardia, palpitations, sweating, blurred vision, incoordination and tremor.

Posthallucinogen perception disorder (flashbacks)
Perceptual changes may be re-experienced years after regular hallucinogen use has ended. This may lead to panic disorder, depression and suicide.

Volatile solvents

Psychological dependence can follow prolonged use.

Types and administration
Psychoactive vapours are given off by solvents, adhesives, petrol, paint, paint thinners, typewriter correction fluid and

some cleaning agents. These substances may be inhaled directly or from containers such as plastic bags (glue sniffing).

Actions

Psychological actions include apathy, belligerence, impaired judgement and euphoria. The physical effects of intoxication include dizziness, nystagmus, blurred vision, incoordination, slurred speech, unsteady gait, lethargy, decreased reflexes, tremor and muscle weakness. High doses may cause stupor, leading to coma.

Schizophrenia, delusional disorders and schizoaffective disorders

....

Schizophrenia and delusional disorders are psychotic disorders in which there may be a lack of contact with reality, for example indicated by the presence of delusions, hallucinations and lack of insight. Schizoaffective disorders are psychotic disorders that have an intermediate position between schizophrenia and mood disorders.

....

SCHIZOPHRENIA
Clinical features

Characteristic features include one or more of the following:

- Changes in thinking
- Changes in perception
- Blunted or inappropriate affect
- A reduced level of social functioning.

Cognitive functions are usually intact in the early stages.

Schneiderian first-rank symptoms
In the absence of organic pathology the presence of any of these symptoms is indicative, though not pathognomonic, of schizophrenia:

- Auditory hallucinations: voices repeating thoughts out loud; voices discussing the subject in the third person; a running commentary
- Thought insertion
- Thought withdrawal
- Thought broadcasting
- Made feelings, impulses and actions
- Somatic passivity
- Delusional perception.

Other ICD-10 symptoms

The following are also not pathognomonic:

- Other persistent delusions
- Persistent hallucinations in any modality, when accompanied by either fleeting or half-formed delusions without clear affective content
- Persistent overvalued ideas
- Breaks or interpolations in the train of thought, which can result in incoherence or irrelevant speech and neologisms
- Catatonic behaviour
- Negative symptoms which typically occur in chronic schizophrenia, including marked apathy, poverty of speech, lack of drive, slowness, and blunting or incongruity of affect. They usually result in social withdrawal and lowered social performance. (Positive symptoms typically occur in acute schizophrenia and include delusions, hallucinations and interference with thoughts)
- A significant and consistent change in the overall quality of some aspects of personal behaviour, manifest as loss of interest, aimlessness, idleness, a self-absorbed attitude and social withdrawal.

DSM-IV criteria

A. *Characteristic symptoms*: At least two of the following, each present for a significant portion of time during a 1-month period (or less, if successfully treated):
   - Delusions
   - Hallucinations
   - Disorganized speech
   - Grossly disorganized or catatonic behaviour
   - Negative symptoms (i.e. affective flattening, alogia or avolition).

If the delusions are bizarre or the hallucinations consist of either a voice keeping up a running commentary on the patient's behaviour or thoughts, or two or more voices conversing with each other, then Criterion A is sufficient to make a DSM-IV diagnosis of schizophrenia. Otherwise, the following criteria are also required.

B. *Social/occupational dysfunction:* In the case of adult onset, for a significant portion of the time since onset at least one major area of social/occupational functioning is markedly below the level achieved before onset of the illness. These areas include:

- Work
- Interpersonal relations
- Self-care.

In the case of onset during childhood or adolescence, there is a failure to achieve the expected level of achievement in the following areas:

- Interpersonal
- Academic
- Occupational.

C. *Duration:* Continuous signs of the disturbance persist for at least 6 months, including at least 1 month of symptoms (or less if successfully treated) that meet Criterion A and that may include periods of prodromal or residual symptoms.

D. *Exclude schizoaffective disorder and mood disorder.*

E. *Exclude substance-related disorder and general medical conditions.*

F. *Relationship to a pervasive developmental disorder:* If there is a history of autistic disorder or another pervasive developmental disorder, the additional diagnosis of schizophrenia is made only if prominent delusions or hallucinations are also present for at least a month (or less, if successfully treated).

Classification

The classification of the World Health Organization includes a number of major ICD-10 subtypes. Based first on psychological studies (Liddle PF. The symptoms of chronic schizophrenia: a re-examination of the positive-negative dichotomy. *British Journal of Psychiatry* 1987; 151:145–151) and then neuroimaging with positron emission tomography (Liddle PF et al. Patterns of cerebral blood flow in schizophrenia. *British Journal of Psychiatry* 1992; 160:179–186), Liddle has classified schizophrenia into three dimensions that correspond to changed metabolic activity in different parts of the brain. A neurodevelopmental classification has also been proposed based on the hypothesis that schizophrenia has a neurodevelopmental origin (Murray RM et al. A neurodevelopmental approach to the classification of schizophrenia. *Schizophrenia Bulletin* 1992; 18:319-333.)

ICD-10 subtypes

- *Paranoid schizophrenia* is dominated by the presence of paranoid symptoms, e.g.:
  - Delusions of persecution
  - Delusions of reference
  - Delusions of exalted birth or of having a special mission
  - Delusions of bodily change
  - Delusions of jealousy
  - Hallucinatory voices of a threatening nature, or that issue commands to the patient
  - Non-verbal auditory hallucinations, e.g. laughing, whistling and humming
  - Hallucinations in other modalities
- *Hebephrenic schizophrenia* is typified by:
  - Irresponsible and unpredictable behaviour
  - Rambling and incoherent speech
  - Affective changes, including an incongruous affect and shallow mood, often with giggling and fatuousness
  - Poorly organized delusions
  - Fleeting and fragmentary hallucinations
- *Catatonic schizophrenia* is dominated by the presence of catatonic symptoms
- *Simple schizophrenia* is characterized by an insidious onset of decline in functioning, both socially and at work or in education. Negative symptoms develop without the prior occurrence of positive symptoms
- *Residual or chronic schizophrenia* is preceded by one of the above types and is characterized by negative symptoms.

DSM-IV subtypes

- *Paranoid type:*
  - Preoccupation with one or more delusions or frequent auditory hallucinations
  - None of the following is prominent:
    - Disorganized speech
    - Disorganized behaviour
    - Catatonic behaviour
    - Flat affect
    - Inappropriate affect

- *Disorganized type:*
  - Disorganized speech is prominent
  - Disorganized behaviour is prominent
  - Flat or inappropriate affect is prominent
  - The criteria for the catatonic type are not met
- *Catatonic type:* at least two of the following dominate the clinical picture:
  - Motor immobility, as evidenced by catalepsy (including waxy flexibility) or stupor
  - Excessive motor activity (which is apparently purposeless and not influenced by external stimuli)
  - Extreme negativism or mutism
  - Peculiarities of voluntary movement as evidenced by posturing, stereotyped movements, prominent mannerisms, or prominent grimacing
  - Echolalia or echopraxia
- *Undifferentiated type:* symptoms meet Criterion A for DSM-IV schizophrenia, but the criteria for the paranoid, disorganized and catatonic types are not met.
- *Residual type:*
  - The following are absent:
    - Prominent delusions
    - Prominent hallucinations
    - Disorganized speech
    - Grossly disorganized behaviour
    - Catatonic behaviour
  - There is continued evidence of the disturbance, as indicated by the presence of negative symptoms or at least two of the symptoms that meet Criterion A for DSM-IV schizophrenia, present in an attenuated form (e.g. odd beliefs, unusual perceptual experiences).

Liddle's classification (see Figure 5.1)

- *Psychomotor poverty syndrome* is characterized by poverty of speech, flatness of affect and decreased spontaneous movement. It is associated with underactivity in the dominant dorsolateral prefrontal cortex, a region maximally activated in normal subjects during self-generated mental activity.
- *Disorganization syndrome* is characterized by disorders of the form of thought and inappropriate affect. It is associated with excessive activity in the non-dominant

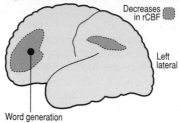

(a) **Psychomotor poverty**

Decreases in rCBF

Left lateral

Word generation

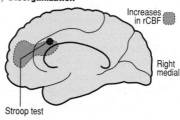

(b) **Disorganization**

Increases in rCBF

Right medial

Stroop test

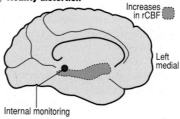

(c) **Reality distortion**

Increases in rCBF

Left medial

Internal monitoring

Figure 5.1
Liddle's classification. **(a)** Locus of maximal activation of the prefrontal cortex during the internal generation of words in normal subjects superimposed on the areas of decreased cortical blood flow associated with psychomotor poverty in schizoprenia. **(b)** Locus of maximal activation of the anterior cingulate cortex during performance of the Stroop test superimposed on the area of increased cortical blood flow associated with disorganization in schizophrenia. **(c)** Locus of maximal activation of the parahippocampal gyrus during the internal monitoring of eye movements superimposed on the area of increased medial temporal blood flow associated with reality distortion in schizophrenia. (Reproduced with permission from Puri BK, Laking PJ, Treasaden IH 1996 Textbook of psychiatry. Edinburgh: Churchill Livingstone.)

anterior cingulate cortex at a site that has been implicated in attention tasks involving the suppression of inappropriate mental activity.
- *Reality distortion syndrome* is characterized by delusions and hallucinations. It is associated with increased activity in the dominant medial temporal lobe, normal functioning of which is involved in internal monitoring; abnormality in this region would be consistent with the patient failing to recognize internally generated mental acts as such.

Neurodevelopmental classification
- In **congenital schizophrenia** the abnormality is present at birth and may be caused by a genetic predisposition and/or an environmental insult. Patients are more likely to have minor physical abnormalities, to show abnormal personality or social impairment in childhood, to present early, to exhibit negative symptoms, and to show morphological brain changes and cognitive impairment. They are more likely to be male and to have a poor outcome.
- Patients with **adult-onset schizophrenia** are likely to exhibit positive symptoms, including schneiderian first-rank symptoms, and mood changes.
- Patients with **late-onset schizophrenia** usually present over the age of 60 and have good premorbid intellectual and occupational functioning. It is more common in females and is often associated with auditory and visual sensory deprivation. Organic brain dysfunction is often found.

Epidemiology
Incidence
Fifteen to 30 new cases per 100 000 of the population per year.

Point prevalence
This is 0.5–1% of the population.

Lifetime risk
Approximately 1%.

Age of onset
Usually between 15 and 45 years. Both mean and median age of onset are earlier in men.

Sex ratio
Equal.

Marriage
Higher incidence in those who are not married. (People with schizophrenia less likely to marry and less likely to have children.)

Social class
Commonest in social classes IV and V because of **social drift**, in which patients drift downwards socially owing to the illness.

Aetiology

Predisposing factors
These include genetic factors (family, twin and adoption studies), prenatal factors (higher incidence in late winter and early spring births, particularly in cases of maternal viral infection), perinatal factors (obstetric complications commoner) and personality (schizotypal personality disorder is commoner in first-degree relatives).

Precipitating factors
Psychosocial stresses (life events) have been suggested.

Perpetuating factors
These include social factors (e.g. poverty of social milieu is associated with increased negative symptoms in chronic schizophrenia) and the patient's family if there is high expressed emotion (relatives make critical comments and become over-involved emotionally).

Mediating factors
These may include neurotransmitters (the dopamine hypothesis, which suggests central dopaminergic hyper-activity in the mesolimbic–mesocortical system; central serotonergic dysfunction; central glutamergic dysfunction), neuronal membrane phospholipid abnormalities, neuro-

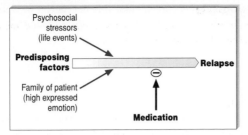

Figure 5.2
The interaction of predisposing factors psychosocial stressors, high expressed emotion and the modifying action of medication. (Reproduced with permission from Puri BK, Laking PJ, Treasaden IH 1996 Textbook of psychiatry. Edinburgh: Churchill Livingstone.)

degeneration, psychoneuroimmunological and psychoneuroendocrinological factors.

These factors interact, as shown in Figure 5.2.

Management

Hospitalization

It is essential to admit those with acute schizophrenic symptoms for investigations and treatment. In addition to routine investigations (see Chapter 1), in the case of first presentation with auditory hallucinations in the elderly, tests of hearing and vision should be carried out, as sensory deprivation is an important cause of these symptoms in this age group. Patients with chronic schizophrenia should be admitted for relapses, but can otherwise often be maintained in the community or in sheltered accommodation. After discharge, regular follow-up appointments with a psychiatrist and, particularly for those with chronic schizophrenia, a community psychiatric nurse, are required.

Drug treatment

Antipsychotic (neuroleptic) drugs are used. Acute schizophrenic (positive) symptoms respond better than chronic (negative) symptoms to typical antipsychotics (e.g. chlorpromazine). Chronic symptoms respond better to atypical (e.g. clozapine and risperidone) than to typical antipsychotics.

Depot antipsychotic preparations can be used for maintenance treatment and improved compliance.

Parkinsonian extrapyramidal side effects can be treated with antimuscarinic (anticholinergic) drugs (e.g. benzhexol and procyclidine).

Recent evidence suggests that the fatty acid EPA (eicosapentaenoic acid) may have a beneficial antipsychotic action for both positive and negative symptoms.

Electroconvulsive therapy (ECT)

This is used to treat cases of catatonic stupor.

Social milieu

In chronic schizophrenia poverty of the social milieu should be reduced using **social skills training**, in which group psychotherapeutic methods are used to teach patients how to interact appropriately with other people, and **occupational therapy**, which teaches useful skills for living outside hospital.

Expressed emotion

For those exposed to high expressed emotion **family therapy** can be offered. If this is not possible or unsuccessful, it may be better for the patient not to live with their family but in a **staffed hostel** instead.

Sheltered workshops

These allow patients to learn a useful skill and gain a sense of achievement.

Prognosis

Approximately 25% show good clinical and social recovery and less than 50% have a poor long-term outcome.

Factors associated with a good prognosis include:

- Female gender
- Having a relative with bipolar mood disorder
- No cognitive impairment
- No ventricular enlargement.

DELUSIONAL (PARANOID) DISORDERS

The core feature of these disorders is the development of a delusion or delusional system which is usually persistent, sometimes lifelong, and does not have an identifiable organic basis. Occasional or transitory auditory hallucinations may occur, particularly in elderly patients.

Epidemiology
Point prevalence
Around 0.03% of the population.

Lifetime risk
This is 0.05–0.1%.

Age of onset
Usually between 40 and 55 years.

Sex ratio
Slightly commoner in females.

Capgras' syndrome

A person who is familiar to the patient is believed to have been replaced by a double. It is commoner in women, with the apparently replaced person often being a relative.

Cotard's syndrome

A nihilistic delusional disorder in which, for example, the patient believes their money, friends or body parts do not exist.

Erotomania (de Clérambault's syndrome)

The patient holds the delusional belief that someone else, usually of a higher social or professional status, is in love with them. It is more common in women.

Fregoli's syndrome

The patient believes that a familiar person, who is often believed to be the patient's persecutor, has taken on different appearances.

Induced psychosis (folie à deux)

Two (or more) people who are closely related emotionally share the delusional disorder. One has a genuine psychotic disorder and their delusional system is induced in the other, who may be dependent or less intelligent.

Pathological (delusional) jealousy

The patient holds the delusional belief that his or her spouse or sexual partner is being unfaithful and goes to great lengths to find evidence of this. It is more common in men.

Persecutory (querulant) delusions

Patients suffer from a delusional system in which they believe they are being persecuted.

Management

Because patients hold their beliefs with delusional intensity, and may also be suspicious, the need for treatment should be explained to them with great care and tact. Relatives and other informants should be interviewed at an early stage. If the patient or others are at risk, hospitalization should be arranged; if voluntary admission is refused then compulsory admission is required. All staff involved should try to establish a good rapport with the patient. If an organic cause, psychoactive substance use, schizophrenia or a mood disorder is found, then this should be treated. If no such primary cause is found antipsychotic medication is usually helpful. In the case of induced psychosis geographical separation usually leads to a remission in the person(s) in whom the disorder is induced.

Prognosis

The course of delusional disorders is variable. Some, particularly persecutory delusions, tend to be chronic, but with varying levels of concern with the delusion.

....

SCHIZOAFFECTIVE DISORDERS

These are episodic disorders in which both symptoms of a mood (affective) disorder and schizophrenic symptoms are prominent within the same episode of illness, either simultaneously or within a few days of each other (ICD-10).

Management

Acute schizophrenic and manic symptoms are treated with antipsychotic drugs, whereas depressive symptoms are treated with antidepressants and/or ECT.

Prognosis

This is probably between those of mood disorders and schizophrenia.

6 Mood disorders

....

In these disorders, which include depressive episodes, bipolar mood disorder and persistent mood disorders, there is a disturbance of mood that is not secondary to organic causes, psychoactive substance use or another psychiatric disorder such as schizophrenia or schizoaffective disorder.

....

DEPRESSIVE EPISODE
Clinical features

Characteristic features of a depressive episode include depression of mood, anhedonia, reduced attention and concentration, ideas of guilt and worthlessness, lowered self-esteem and reduced energy, which in turn causes tiredness and reduced activity. In turn, these can lead to hopelessness and a belief that life is not worth living, which can cause suicidal thoughts. Biological symptoms occur frequently (Table 6.1); the types of sleep disturbance that may occur in depressive episodes are shown diagrammatically in Figure 6.1.

Table 6.1 Biological symptoms of depression

↓ Appetite
↓ Weight
Constipation
Sleep disturbance, such as:
   Early morning wakening
   Initial insomnia
   Broken sleep
Diurnal variation of mood
↓ Libido
Amenorrhoea

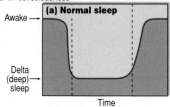

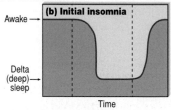

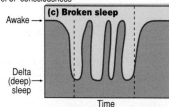

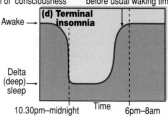

Figure 6.1
Types of sleep disturbance in depressive episodes. (**a**) Normal sleep (**b**) Initial insomnia. (**c**) Broken sleep. (**d**) Early morning wakening (also known as terminal insomnia). Reproduced with permission from Puri BK, Laking PJ, Treasaden IH 1996 Textbook of psychiatry. Edinburgh: Churchill Livingstone.)

Mental state examination

Appearance

Depressive facies include downturned eyes, sagging of the corners of the mouth and a vertical furrow between the eyebrows. There is typically poor eye contact. There may be direct evidence of weight loss, with the patient appearing emaciated and dehydrated. Indirect evidence of recent weight loss may be indicated by the clothing appearing to be too large. Evidence of poor self-care and general neglect may include an unkempt appearance, poor personal hygiene and dirty clothing.

Behaviour

Psychomotor retardation typically occurs.

Speech

The patient's speech is typically slow, with long delays before questions are answered.

Mood

The mood is low and sad, with feelings of hopelessness. The future seems bleak. Anxiety, irritability and agitation may also occur. The patient may complain of reduced energy and drive, and an inability to feel enjoyment (anhedonia). There is a loss of interest in normal activities and hobbies.

Thought content

Pessimistic thoughts occur concerning the past, present and future. Suicidal and homicidal thoughts may occur and should be checked for. Obsessions may occur secondary to depression.

Abnormal beliefs and interpretation of events

Ideas or delusions of a hypochondriacal or nihilistic nature may be present.

Abnormal experiences

In severe depressive episodes auditory hallucinations may occur which are typically in the second person and derogatory in content.

Cognition

Concentration is characteristically poor.

DSM-IV criteria for major depressive episode

A. At least five of the following symptoms have been present during the same 2-week period and represent a change from previous functioning; at least one of the symptoms is either (1) or (2):

  (1) Depressed mood most of the day, nearly every day, as indicated by either subjective report (e.g. feels sad or empty) or observation by others (e.g. appears tearful). In children and adolescents this can be irritable mood.

  (2) Markedly diminished interest or pleasure in all, or almost all, activities most of the day, nearly every day.

  (3) Significant weight loss when not dieting or weight gain (e.g. a change of > 5% body weight in a month), or a decrease or increase in appetite nearly every day. In children consider failure to make expected weight gains.

  (4) Insomnia or hypersomnia nearly every day.

  (5) Psychomotor agitation or retardation (observable by others) nearly every day.

  (6) Fatigue or loss of energy nearly every day.

  (7) Feelings of worthlessness or excessive or inappropriate guilt (which may be delusional) nearly every day.

  (8) Diminished ability to think or concentrate, or indecisiveness, nearly every day.

  (9) Recurrent thoughts of death (not just fear of dying), recurrent suicidal ideation without a specific plan, or a suicide attempt or a specific plan for committing suicide.

B. Exclude a mixed episode (in which a manic episode also occurs).

C. The symptoms cause clinically significant distress or impairment in social, occupational or other important areas of functioning.

D. The symptoms are not caused either by a direct physiological action of a substance (e.g. a drug of abuse, or medication), or by a general medical condition (e.g. hypothyroidism).

E. The symptoms are not better accounted for by bereavement.

Differentiation from bereavement

The duration of a normal grief reaction varies in different cultures. In DSM-IV a diagnosis of major depressive episode/disorder is generally not given unless the symptoms are still present 2 months after the loss. In differentiating a depressive episode (major depressive episode in DSM-IV) from a normal grief reaction, the following DSM-IV criteria are also held to be more likely to point to a diagnosis of a (major) depressive episode:

- Guilt about things other than actions taken or not taken by the survivor at the time of death
- Thoughts of death other than the survivor feeling that he or she would be better off dead, or should have died with the deceased
- Morbid preoccupation with worthlessness
- Marked psychomotor retardation
- Prolonged and marked functional impairment
- Hallucinations other than thinking that one hears the voice of, or transiently sees the image of, the deceased.

Atypical types of depression

Depressive stupor

This is rare these days because of effective treatment.

Masked depression

Depressed patients may present with somatic or other complaints instead of a depressed mood. They may somatize their depressed mood because of cultural factors, or they may not be able to articulate their emotions, as in the case of patients with severe learning disability and elderly patients with dementia. In such cases the presence of biological symptoms of depression is particularly helpful in making the diagnosis. In the case of patients with learning disability diurnal variations in abnormal behaviour may be observed and may mirror diurnal variations in mood.

Seasonal affective disorder (SAD)

The onset of depressive episodes is related to a particular time or season. For example, untreated depressive episodes may regularly start in autumn or winter and end in spring or summer. The onset of bipolar disorders may also be seasonal. During depressive episodes patients with SAD often exhibit carbohydrate craving, hypersomnia and weight gain. Excluded from this category are cases in which there is a clearly distinguished seasonal psychosocial stressor, e.g. becoming depressed each winter because of regular winter unemployment.

Agitated depression
This occurs in the elderly.

Investigations

In addition to routine investigations (see Chapter 1), in the case of first presentation with auditory hallucinations in the elderly tests of hearing and vision should be carried out, as sensory deprivation is an important cause of these symptoms in this age group.

The physical examination should include a careful inspection for any evidence of self-harm, such as scars on the wrists.

Epidemiology

Incidence
In males, 80–200 new cases per 100 000 population per year. In females, 250–7800 new cases per 100 000 population per year.

Point prevalence
In the west, 1.8–3.2% of males, and 2.0–9.3% of females. The point prevalence of depressive symptoms in western populations is up to 20%.

Lifetime risk
In the general population of western countries 5–12% in males and 9–26% in females.

Age of onset
On average, around the late 30s. However, it can start anywhere from childhood to old age.

Sex ratio
Commoner in females.

Marriage

Higher incidence in those who are not married, including the divorced and separated.

Social class

Higher incidence in working-class, rather than middle-class, women and in women who:

- Have three or more children under the age of 14 to look after
- Do not work outside the home
- Do not have somebody to confide in, that is, there is a lack of intimacy
- Lost their own mother before the age of 11, through death or separation.

Aetiology

This is considered under bipolar disorder (below). The reasons for the increased incidence and prevalence in females are not known. Possibilities suggested include:

- Women may be more likely to admit to feeling depressed.
- Depression may be underdiagnosed in men, who may be more likely to engage in excessive alcohol consumption and therefore be diagnosed as suffering from psychoactive substance use disorder rather than depression.
- Women may suffer from greater stresses, such as childbirth and hormonal effects (menarche, premenstrual syndrome and menopause).

Management

Hospitalization

Less severe episodes can be treated by GPs in the community or by psychiatrists in outpatient clinics. Patients suffering from severe episodes should be admitted for inpatient treatment. In the case of severe life-threatening features, such as suicide risk or poor food and fluid intake, this may require compulsory admission against the will of the patient.

Drug treatment

Antidepressant medication is the mainstay of treatment for moderate and severe depressive episodes. Mild depressive symptoms can also benefit from such treatment.

Electroconvulsive therapy (ECT)

This may be used as a first line of treatment in the following relatively rare conditions:

- Very low fluid intake, resulting in oliguria
- Depressive stupor
- A dangerously high risk of suicide.

Mostly, however, ECT is reserved for cases of resistant depression not responding to medication.

Psychosurgery

This is considered only extremely rarely, when all other treatments for severe chronic handicapping depression have failed.

Phototherapy

SAD with an autumn or winter onset can be treated with high-intensity light.

Psychotherapies

The following are available for mild or moderate depression, or following recovery from severe depressive episodes:

- Cognitive therapy
- Group therapy
- Psychoanalytic psychotherapy
- Family therapy
- Marital therapy.

Social milieu

Increased activity and social contact should be encouraged. The development of confiding relationships has a protective function in preventing relapse. Occupational therapy can be useful in enabling inpatients to learn to cope with life skills.

Prognosis

The outcome in general is better the greater the length of follow-up. The risk of relapse is reduced if antidepressant medication is continued for 6 months after the end of the depressive episode. Overall, the suicide rate is around 9%.

....

BIPOLAR DISORDER

In DSM-IV the essential feature of bipolar disorder is the occurrence of at least one episode of mania (or hypomania), whereas in ICD-10 there must be a history of at least two episodes of mood disturbance, at least one of which should have been mania (or hypomania) (see Figure 6.2).

Clinical features of mania

There is elevation of mood, increased energy, overactivity, pressure of speech, reduced sleep, loss of normal social and sexual inhibitions, and poor attention and concentration. The elevated mood may manifest itself as euphoria, but sometimes patients can instead be irritable and angry. The patient may overspend, start unrealistic projects, be sexually promiscuous, and, if irritable or angry, be inappropriately aggressive. Neglect of eating, drinking and personal hygiene may result in dangerous states of dehydration and self-neglect.

Mental state examination

Appearance

The patient may be flamboyantly dressed. In severe cases signs of self-neglect may be present (e.g. appearing unkempt and dehydrated).

Behaviour

Overactivity is characteristic. The patient may not sit still.

Speech

There is pressure of speech. Flight of ideas is common in severe mania, with the connections between topics being based, for example, on chance relationships, verbal associations, clang associations, and distracting stimuli.

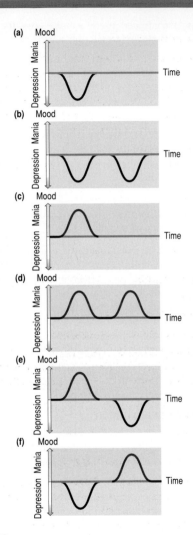

Figure 6.2
Classification of mood disorders by DSM-IV and ICD-10. **(a)** Depressive episode. **(b)** Recurrent depressive episodes. **(c)** Bipolar disorder in DSM-IV, manic episode in ICD-10. **(d-f)** Bipolar disorder in both DSM-IV and ICD-10. (Reproduced with permission from Puri BK, Laking PJ, Treasaden IH 1996 Textbook of psychiatry. Edinburgh: Churchill Livingstone.)

Mood
Euphoria or irritability occur.

Thought content and abnormal beliefs
The patient has an inflated view of his or her own importance and expansive and grandiose ideas about the significance of his or her opinions and work. These may develop into delusions. Irritability and suspiciousness may develop into delusions of persecution.

Abnormal experiences
Subjective hyperacusis and auditory or visual hallucinations may occur.

Cognitions
Attention and concentration are poor.

Insight
Insight is characteristically absent.

Subtypes of mania

Hypomania
This is a lesser degree of mania (ICD-10).

Mania without psychotic symptoms

Mania with psychotic symptoms
Delusions and hallucinations occur in addition to the other clinical features of mania. These may include schneiderian first-rank symptoms.

Manic stupor
Owing to effective treatment this is rare.

DSM-IV criteria for manic episode

A. A distinct period of abnormally and persistently elevated, expansive or irritable mood, lasting at least 1 week (or less if hospitalization is necessary).

B. During this period at least three of the following symptoms have persisted (at least four if the mood is only irritable), and have been present to a significant degree:

    (1) Inflated self-esteem or grandiosity
    (2) Decreased need for sleep

(3) More talkative than usual, or pressure to keep talking
(4) Flight of ideas or subjective experience that thoughts are racing
(5) Distractibility (i.e. attention too easily drawn to unimportant or irrelevant external stimuli)
(6) Increase in goal-directed activity (either socially, at work or school, or sexually) or psychomotor agitation
(7) Excessive involvement in pleasurable activities that have a high potential for painful consequences (e.g. engaging in unrestrained buying sprees, sexual indiscretions or foolish business investments)

C. Exclude a mixed episode (in which a major depressive episode also occurs).

D. The mood disturbance causes any of the following:

- Marked impairment in occupational functioning
- Marked impairment in usual social activities
- Marked impairment in relationships with others
- Hospitalization is necessary to prevent harm to self or others
- Psychotic features.

E. The symptoms are not caused either by a direct physiological action of a substance (e.g. a drug of abuse, medication or other treatment) or by a general medical condition (e.g. hyperthyroidism).

DSM-IV criteria for hypomanic episode

A. A distict period persitently elevated, expansive or irritable mood, lasting throughout at least 4 days, that is clearly different from the usual non-depressed mood.

B. During this period at least three of the following symptoms have persisted (at least four if the mood is only irritable) and have been present to a significant degree:

(1) Inflated self-esteem or grandiosity
(2) Decreased need for sleep
(3) More talkative than usual, or pressure to keep talking

(4) Flight of ideas or subjective experience that thoughts are racing

(5) Distractibility (i.e. attention too easily drawn to unimportant or irrelevant external stimuli)

(6) Increase in goal-directed activity (either socially, at work or school, or sexually) or psychomotor agitation

(7) Excessive involvment in pleasurable activities that have a high potential for painful consequences (e.g. engaging in unrestrained buying sprees, sexual indiscretions or foolish business investments).

C. The episode is associated with an unequivocal change in functioning that is uncharacteristic of the person when not symptomatic.

D. The mood disturbance and change in functioning are observable by others.

E. The episode is not severe enough to cause marked impairment in social or occupational functioning, or to necessitate hospitalization, and there are no psychotic features.

F. The symptoms are not caused either by a direct physiological action of a substance (e.g. a drug of abuse, medication or other treatment), or by a general medical condition (e.g. hyperthyroidism).

Epidemiology of bipolar disorder

Point prevalence
In the US 0.4–1.2% of the adult population.

Lifetime risk
In the US 0.6–1.1% in the adult population.

Age of onset
On average around the mid-20s, but it can start for the first time in old age. In adolescence it may be mistaken for schizophrenia.

Sex ratio
Equal.

Social class
Commoner in the upper social classes.

Aetiology of depressive episodes and bipolar disorders

Predisposing factors

These include genetic factors (family, twin and adoption studies) and personality (cyclothymic or cycloid personality disorder may predispose to bipolar disorder).

Precipitating factors

These include psychosocial stresses (life events) and physical illnesses (e.g. viral infections are associated with depression).

Perpetuating and mediating factors

These include social factors, psychological factors (e.g. cognitive dysfunction), the patient's family (high expressed emotion at home is associated with an increased risk of relapse of depression), neurotransmitters (changes in central functional noradrenaline and serotonin), psychoneuroendocrinological factors, water and electrolyte changes, and photic changes.

Management

Hospitalization

A (hypo)manic patient should be admitted. If suffering from self-neglect and dehydration, these should be treated in addition to the manic symptoms.

Drug treatment

Antipsychotic drugs such as haloperidol and chlorpromazine (given intramuscularly if necessary) act rapidly and are the mainstay of the treatment of acute mania.

Lithium salts (lithium carbonate and lithium citrate) are used in the prophylaxis of mania and, therefore, of bipolar disorder. Lithium has a low therapeutic ratio and therefore regular plasma level monitoring is essential to keep the concentration between 0.4 and 1.0 mmol/l (measured 12 hours after the last dose). Urea and electrolytes and thyroid function need to be monitored regularly during lithium theraphy. If the disorder is resistant to lithium prophylactic **carbamazepine** can be tried, with regular plasma level monitoring.

Electroconvulsive therapy (ECT)
This is used in treating rare cases of manic stupor.

Family therapy
This may be needed if the patient is subjected to a high level of expressed emotion.

Prognosis

The prognosis of bipolar disorder is much better in those who regularly take prophylactic medication (lithium salts or carbamazepine).

PERSISTENT MOOD DISORDERS

These are persistent and usually fluctuating disorders of mood in which individual episodes are rarely if ever sufficiently severe to warrant being described as hypomanic, or even mild depressive episodes (ICD-10).

Cyclothymia

There is a persistent instability of mood, involving numerous periods of mild depression and mild elation, usually developing early in adult life and pursuing a chronic course (ICD-10).

Lifetime risk
This is 0.4–3.5%.

Sex ratio
Equal.

First-degree biological relatives
There are more likely than the general population to suffer from depressive episodes and bipolar disorder.

Management
If patients come to medical attention they may respond to lithium and/or individual or group psychotherapy. Hospitalization is not usually indicated.

Dysthymia (depressive neurosis)

There is a chronic depression of mood which does not fulfil the criteria for recurrent depressive disorder. Patients brood and complain, sleep badly and feel inadequate, but are usually able to cope with the basic demands of everyday life (ICD-10).

It is commoner in the first-degree biological relatives of patients with a history of depressive episodes than in the general population.

Sex ratio

Probably commoner in females.

Management

In severe cases treatment with antidepressants, individual psychotherapy or cognitive therapy may be helpful. Hospitalization is not usually indicated unless the patient is suicidal.

Neurotic, stress-related and somatoform disorders

In ICD-10 neurotic, stress-related and somatoform disorders are brought together in one overall group because of their historical association with the concept of neurosis and the association of a substantial proportion of these disorders with psychological causation. Mixtures of symptoms are common, particularly coexistent depression and anxiety.

AGORAPHOBIA

Clinical features

Agoraphobia consists of a cluster of anxiety-causing phobias which embraces fears of leaving home (e.g. fear of entering shops), crowds, public places, and travelling alone on public transport. These cause the patient to become housebound. The lack of an immediately available exit is a key feature of many of these agoraphobic situations (ICD-10).

Epidemiology

Age of onset

Variable, but often starts in the 20s or 30s.

Sex ratio

More common in females.

Management

The treatment of choice is behaviour therapy, involving exposure combined with anxiety management. Short-term anxiolytics and antidepressants for any associated depressive symptoms may be considered: monoamine oxidase inhibitors (MAOIs) and reversible inhibitors of monoamine oxidase type A (RIMAs) may be particularly helpful.

Prognosis

In the absence of effective treatment agoraphobia typically persists for years, though usually fluctuating.

SOCIAL PHOBIA
Clinical features

The phobias centre on a fear of scrutiny by other people in comparatively small groups (as opposed to crowds), leading to an avoidance of social situations, such as eating in public, public speaking, and encounters with the opposite sex (ICD-10).

Epidemiology
Age of onset
Often begins in adolescence.

Sex ratio
Equal.

Management

The treatment of choice is behaviour therapy, involving exposure combined with anxiety management.

Prognosis

It is usually chronic, if untreated, and may be exacerbated if performance in the phobic situations is worsened because of anxiety.

SPECIFIC (ISOLATED) PHOBIA
Clinical features

The phobias are restricted to highly specific situations, e.g. proximity to animals, heights, thunder, darkness, flying, closed spaces, eating certain foods, dentistry, and the fear of exposure to specific diseases such as AIDS and radiation sickness (ICD-10). Contact with the triggering situation may lead to panic.

Epidemiology
Age of onset
Usually starts in childhood or early adult life.

Sex ratio
More common in females.

Management

The treatment of choice is behaviour therapy, involving exposure combined with anxiety management.

Prognosis

In the absence of effective treatment specific phobias can persist for years.

....

PANIC DISORDER
Clinical features

There are recurrent attacks of severe anxiety (panic) which are not restricted to any particular situation and which are therefore unpredictable (ICD-10). Symptoms include a sudden onset of palpitations, chest pain, choking, dizziness, sweating, trembling; depersonalization or derealization; and a secondary fear of dying, going mad or losing control. Attacks tend to last for only a few minutes but during them the anxiety and autonomic symptoms build up quickly, often leading to a hurried exit from where the patient is.

Exclude organic causes such as hypoglycaemic episodes, hyperthyroidism and phaeochromocytoma. Panic disorder may be secondary to depressive episodes.

Epidemiology
Sex ratio
More common in females.

Management
Supportive measures
The patient should be reassured and the causes of individual symptoms, e.g. palpitations, should be given to allay unnecessary worry.

Drug treatment

Antidepressants (e.g. imipramine) are effective in treating panic disorder, whether or not there is an underlying depressive disorder. Anxiolytics, including buspirone and benzodiazepines, can be used for the short-term management of anxiety disorders.

Cognitive therapy

In patients worried about physical consequences of anxiety symptoms, e.g. that palpitations are related to heart disease, the symptoms are induced voluntarily, e.g. by hyperventilation or exercise, and their nature is explained.

GENERALIZED ANXIETY DISORDER
Clinical features

Generalized and persistent anxiety that is not restricted to, or even strongly predominating in, any particular environmental situation, i.e. it is free-floating (ICD-10). Symptoms can result from sympathetic overactivity, increased muscle tension and hyperventilation (see Figure 7.1), and commonly include a continuous feeling of nervousness, trembling, muscular tension, sweating, light-headedness, palpitations, dizziness, dry mouth, epigastric discomfort, and increased frequency and urgency of micturition. Sleep disturbance may occur, typically with initial insomnia while the patient lies in bed worrying, and broken sleep thereafter.

Epidemiology
Sex ratio
More common in females.

Management

This is as for panic disorder. Relaxation training may help, and the patient can be taught to rebreathe from a bag or practise controlled breathing during hyperventilation. If there is no response to the drug treatments mentioned above, β-adrenergic antagonists can be considered.

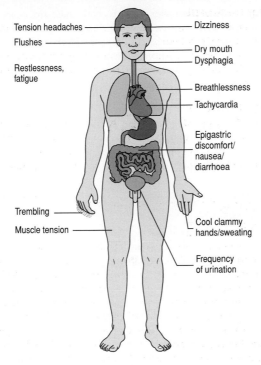

Figure 7.1
Somatic clinical features of generalized anxiety disorder. (Reproduced with permission from Puri BK, Laking PJ, Treasaden IH 1996 Textbook of psychiatry. Edinburgh: Churchill Livingstone.)

Prognosis

This is variable, although the course tends to be chronic and fluctuating.

OBSESSIVE–COMPULSIVE DISORDER
Clinical features

Recurrent obsessional thoughts and/or compulsive acts occur which are recognized as being one's own and which are unsuccessfully resisted, although in long-standing cases the resistance may be minimal. Obsessional thoughts are almost always distressing, e.g. because they are violent, obscene or senseless, and compulsive acts or rituals are not inherently enjoyable or useful, for example handwashing. Depressive symptoms commonly coexist, sometimes as a result of a primary depressive disorder.

Epidemiology

Age of onset
Usually starts in childhood or early adult life.

Sex ratio
Equal.

Management

Supportive measures
The patient should be reassured that 'madness' is not imminent and the causes of individual symptoms should be given.

Drug treatment
Antidepressants that inhibit serotonin reuptake (e.g. selective serotonin reuptake inhibitors (SSRIs) and clomipramine) are often effective.

Behaviour therapy
In cases of compulsive acts behaviour therapy, involving exposure to any external cues and response prevention, is usually effective. If obsessional thoughts without compulsions occur, thought-stopping may sometimes be helpful.

Psychosurgery
Psychosurgical procedures, e.g. subcaudate tractotomy, leucotomy and limbic leucotomy, are used only as a last resort in severe intractable cases.

Prognosis

There is a variable course. If no depressive symptoms are present then without treatment the condition is more likely to be chronic.

ACUTE STRESS REACTION
Clinical features

A transient disorder of significant severity develops in a person who has no other mental disorder in response to exceptional physical and/or mental stress (e.g. an accident or a natural catastrophe). It usually subsides within hours or days (ICD-10).

Management

The patient should be allowed to ventilate his or her thoughts and emotions. In severe cases very short-term use only of anxiolytic medication may be needed.

POST-TRAUMATIC STRESS DISORDER
Clinical features

This arises as a delayed and/or protracted response to a stressful event or a situation of an exceptionally threatening or catastrophic nature that is likely to cause pervasive distress in almost anyone (e.g. torture or rape). Episodes of repeated reliving of the trauma in intrusive memories (flashbacks) or dreams may occur against a persisting background of a sense of numbness, emotional blunting, anhedonia, detachment from others and avoidance of anything reminiscent of the trauma (ICD-10). There is usually a state of autonomic hyperarousal (hypervigilance, increased startle reaction and insomnia), and anxiety, depression and alcohol and drug abuse may occur.

Management

Neurological examination is required if there is any possibility of brain injury during the stressful event. Supportive psychotherapy is required and anxiolytic drug treatment may be needed.

Prognosis

In most cases there is recovery within 6 months. In a minority the condition has a chronic course over years and may lead to an enduring personality change.

ADJUSTMENT DISORDERS
Clinical features

These are states of subjective distress and emotional disturbance (e.g. a depressive or anxiety reaction), usually interfering with social functioning and performance, and arising in the period of adaptation to a significant life change or event (e.g. bereavement, separation, migration or serious physical illness) (ICD-10).

Management

Brief psychotherapy enables the patient to adjust to his or her new circumstances.

Prognosis

The symptoms usually do not persist beyond 6 months, except in the case of a prolonged depressive reaction in which a mild depressive state may last up to 2 years.

DISSOCIATIVE (CONVERSION) DISORDERS
Clinical features

There is a partial or complete loss of the normal integration between memories of the past, awareness of identity and immediate sensations, and control of bodily movements, which is psychogenic in origin, being closely associated in time with traumatic events, insoluble and intolerable problems or disturbed relationships (ICD-10). Types of dissociative disorder include:

- *Dissociative amnesia*, in which there is amnesia for events that are traumatic or stressful in nature, in the absence of organic brain disorder, intoxication or excessive fatigue
- *Dissociative fugue*, in which, in addition to the features of dissociative amnesia, purposeful travel takes place beyond the everyday range, while basic self-care and simple social interactions are maintained
- *Dissociative stupor*

- *Trance and possession disorders*
- *Dissociative disorders of movement and sensation*, in which there is loss of or interference with movements or loss of sensations in the absence of an organic cause
- *Ganser's syndrome*, characterized by the giving of approximate answers (e.g. when asked how many legs a cow has, the patient may reply 'five', showing that the question is understood), usually together with other dissociative symptoms
- *Multiple personality disorder*, in which two or more distinct and complete personalities appear to exist within one person, with only one being evident at a time.

Management

Reassurance and explanation are important. Abreaction or psychodynamic psychotherapy may enable the patient to work through the original cause.

Prognosis

Dissociative states endured for more than 2 years before presentation to a psychiatrist are often resistant to treatment.

....
SOMATOFORM DISORDERS
Clinical features

There is repeated presentation of physical symptoms, together with persistent requests for medical investigations in spite of repeated negative findings and reassurances from doctors that the symptoms have no physical basis (ICD-10). Types include:

- *Somatization disorder*, in which there are multiple, recurrent and frequently changing physical symptoms, which have usually been present for several years before referral to a psychiatrist
- *Hypochondrial disorder*, in which there is a persistent preoccupation with the possibility of having one or more serious and progressive physical disorders
- *Persistent somatoform pain disorder* (psychogenic pain), in which the patient complains of persistent, severe and

distressing pain which cannot be explained fully medically.

Management

The psychiatric and medical teams need to work closely and give the patient a consistent message. When all investigations have been carried out the patient should be told this and not offered any further ones. Instead, the condition should be patiently explained and reassurance given. If appropriate, other interventions such as anxiety management or antidepressants may be offered.

....

INTERACTION BETWEEN PSYCHIATRIC AND PHYSICAL ILLNESS

Table 7.1 outlines the interactions between psychiatric and physical illness.

Examples of pathophysiological mechanisms that have been proposed for specific medically unexplained symptoms are shown in Figure 7.2.

Table 7.2 gives some examples of the factors that influence a patient's response to a physical illness.

Table 7.1 Interaction between psychiatric and physical illness (Reproduced with permission from Puri BK, Laking PJ, Treasaden IH 1996 Textbook of psychiatry. Edinburgh: Churchill Livingstone.)

Organic mental disorders
Physical illness has direct effect on brain function
- delirium/acute confusional state/organic psychosis, e.g. liver failure
- dementia/chronic organic psychosis
- postoperative psychosis

Maladaptive psychological reactions to illness
Depression, e.g. amputation, mastectomy (owing to loss)
Guilt, e.g. fear of burden on relatives
Anxiety, e.g. before operation, unpleasant procedure
Paranoid reaction, e.g. if deaf, blind
Anger
Denial
Preoccupation with illness
Prolongation of sick role (fewer responsibilities, more attention)

Psychosomatic disease
Multiple (i.e. biopsychosocial) causes
e.g. life events/stress on physically and emotionally vulnerable leads to changes in nervous, endocrine systems etc. and disease, e.g. bereavement may precipitate a heart attack, or stress may precipitate asthma, eczema, peptic ulcer

Psychiatric conditions presenting with physical complaints
Somatic (physical) anxiety symptoms owing to autonomic hyperactivity, e.g. palpitations
Conversion disorders (via voluntary nervous system)
Depression leading to facial pain, constipation, hypochondriacal complaints and delusions, e.g. cancer, VD
Hypochondriacal disorder: excessive concern with health and normal sensations
Somatization disorder
Monosymptomatic hypochondriacal delusions, e.g. delusions of infestation or smell; and other psychotic disorders, e.g. schizophrenia
Munchausen's (hospital addiction) syndrome
Alcoholism leading to liver disease
Self-neglect

Physical conditions presenting with psychiatric complaints
Depressive disorder precipitated by cancer, e.g. of pancreas
Anxiety in hyperthyroidism
Postviral depression, e.g. post hepatitis, glandular fever, influenza

Medical drugs leading to psychiatric complications
e.g. Antihypertensive drugs leading to depression
e.g. Corticosteroids leading to depression, euphoria

Psychiatric drugs leading to medical complications
e.g. Overdoses
e.g. Chlorpromazine leading to jaundice

Coincidental psychiatric and physical disorder

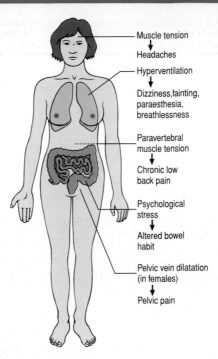

Figure 7.2
Pathophysiological mechanisms proposed for specific medically
unexplained symptoms. (Reproduced with permission from Puri
BK, Laking PJ, Treasaden IH 1996 Textbook of psychiatry.
Edinburgh: Churchill Livingstone)

Table 7.2 Factors influencing the response to a physical illness. (Reproduced with permission from Puri BK, Laking PJ, Treasaden IH 1996 Textbook of psychiatry. Edinburgh: Churchill Livingstone.)

Patient
Personality (e.g. overanxious, obsessional)
Illness behaviour (e.g. at what severity does the patient present)

Illness
Meaning and significance of illness (e.g. cancer)

Social environment
Threat to finances and employment
Welcomed if resolves conflict (e.g. marital)

8   Eating disorders

Two important and well defined eating disorders are outlined in this chapter: anorexia nervosa and bulimia nervosa.

ANOREXIA NERVOSA
Clinical features

This is a disorder characterized by deliberate weight loss, induced and/or sustained by the patient using a number of strategies, including avoiding 'fattening' foods, self-induced vomiting and/or purging, excessive exercise, and using diuretics and/or appetite suppressants. The ICD-10 criterion for body weight is that it is maintained at least 15% below that expected, or that Quetelet's body-mass index (mass $(kg)/[height\ (m)]^2$) is less than or equal to $17.5\ kg/m^2$. The patient has body-image distortion and a dread of fatness. Disorder of the hypothalamic–pituitary–gonadal axis leads, in women, to amenorrhoea (although if taking the oral contraceptive pill breakthrough vaginal bleeding continues to take place) and, in men, to low libido and erectile dysfunction. If the onset is prepubertal in girls, breast development does not take place and there is primary amenorrhoea; in boys the genitals do not develop. Psychiatric symptomatology most commonly associated with anorexia nervosa includes:

- *Obsessive–compulsive behaviour*, e.g. compulsive handwashing and weight checking
- *Anxiety*, particularly related to food and eating
- *Mood disorder*, including depressive episodes (with suicidal thoughts, poor concentration and social withdrawal) and labile mood.

DSM-IV criteria for anorexia nervosa

The four criteria are:

- Refusal to maintain body weight at or above a minimally normal weight for age and height (e.g. weight loss leading to maintenance of body weight < 85% of that expected; or failure to make expected weight gain during period of growth, leading to body weight < 85% of that expected
- Intense fear of gaining weight or becoming fat, even though underweight
- Disturbance in the way in which one's body weight or shape is experienced, undue influence of body weight or shape on self-evaluation, or denial of the seriousness of the current low body weight
- In postmenarchal females amenorrhoea, i.e. the absence of at least three consecutive menstrual cycles. (A woman is considered to have amenorrhoea if her periods occur only following hormone, e.g. oestrogen, administration.)

Restricting type

During the current episode of anorexia nervosa the patient has not regularly engaged in binge-eating or purging behaviour (i.e. self-induced vomiting or the misuse of laxatives, diuretics or enemas).

Binge-eating/purging type

During the current episode of anorexia nervosa the patient has regularly engaged in binge-eating or purging behaviour (i.e. self-induced vomiting or the misuse of laxatives, diuretics or enemas).

Physical examination

Patients appear thin and emaciated. There may be evidence of dehydration, salivary gland swelling, dental caries and perimyolysis. Lanugo hair is often present on the face and back. Axillary and pubic hair are present (cf. hypopituitarism, in which they are absent or scanty). There may be evidence of a poor peripheral circulation (Figure 8.1).

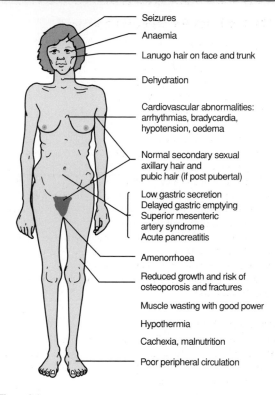

Seizures

Anaemia

Lanugo hair on face and trunk

Dehydration

Cardiovascular abnormalities:
arrhythmias, bradycardia,
hypotension, oedema

Normal secondary sexual
axillary hair and
pubic hair (if post pubertal)

Low gastric secretion
Delayed gastric emptying
Superior mesenteric
artery syndrome
Acute pancreatitis

Amenorrhoea

Reduced growth and risk of
osteoporosis and fractures

Muscle wasting with good power

Hypothermia

Cachexia, malnutrition

Poor peripheral circulation

Figure 8.1
Physical features associated with anorexia nervosa. (Reproduced with
permission from Puri BK, Laking PJ, Treasaden IH 1996 Textbook of
psychiatry. Edinburgh: Churchill Livingstone.)

Investigations

The differential diagnosis of anorexia nervosa (and bulimia
nervosa) is summarized in Table 8.1. Organic causes of
weight loss in young patients should be excluded, e.g.
chronic debilitating diseases, brain tumours, and intestinal
disorders such as Crohn's disease or malabsorption
syndromes. The body weight and height should be carefully
measured. The former acts as a baseline from which to
monitor progress during treatment. Abnormal investigation
results that may be found include the following.

Table 8.1 Differential diagnosis of anorexia nervosa and bulimia nervosa. (Reproduced with permission from Puri BK, Laking PJ, Treasaden IH 1996 Textbook of psychiatry. Edinburgh: Churchill Livingstone.)

Psychiatric	Depression
	Obsessive–compulsive disorder
	Personality disorder
Physical	Chronic debilitating disorders
	Neoplasia
	Thyroid disorder
	Intracranial space-occupying lesions
	Malabsorption syndromes
	Intestinal disorders, including Crohn's disease

Haematological

Leucopenia and mild anaemia are common; thrombocytopenia occurs rarely.

Metabolic

- Metabolic alkalosis ($\uparrow$plasma bicarbonate), hypochloraemia and hypokalaemia secondary to induced vomiting
- $\uparrow$Blood urea nitrogen secondary to dehydration
- Hypercholesterolaemia is common
- Raised liver function tests may occur
- Metabolic acidosis may occur secondary to laxative abuse
- Hypomagnesaemia, $\uparrow$plasma amylase, fasting hypoglycaemia, $\downarrow$plasma zinc and hypercarotenaemia are occasionally seen
- Plasma protein and albumin levels are commonly normal

Plasma hormones

- Thyroxine (T_4) levels are usually in the low-normal range
- $\downarrow T_3$, $\uparrow rT_3$, $\uparrow$basal somatotropin (growth hormone), $\uparrow$cortisol, $\downarrow$oestrogen in females, $\downarrow$testosterone in males, abnormalities of insulin secretion, and abnormal neuroendocrine challenge responses
- In males and females the pattern of secretion of luteinizing hormone (LH) is similar to that seen before or at puberty.

Urine

Picture of dehydration, $\downarrow$GFR, $\downarrow$gonadotropins, $\downarrow$oestrogens.

ECG
Bradycardia, arrhythmias (rare), ↑QT interval, ST depression, T-wave flattening or inversion.

EEG
Fluid and electrolyte disturbances may lead to diffuse abnormalities (metabolic encephalopathy).

Resting energy expenditure
Often significantly reduced.

Structural neuroimaging
Starvation may lead to an increased ventricle-to-brain ratio (VBR).

Epidemiology
Incidence
In the west, 0.4–4 new cases per 100 000 of the population per year. For females aged 15–24 years the incidence is 10–11 new cases per 100 000 per year.

Point prevalence
In UK adolescent schoolgirls and female university students 1–2%. Approximately another 5% exhibit some features but do not reach diagnostic criteria.

Age of onset
Usually in adolescence. The peak age of onset in females is 16–18 years; in males the peak onset is at 12 years.

Sex ratio
At least 90% of those affected are female.

Ethnicity
Rare in the non-white populations of both western and non-western countries.

Social class
Commoner in social classes I and II.

Occupation
There is a higher prevalence in occupations concerned with body weight, e.g. modelling and ballet students.

Aetiology

Predisposing factors
Genetic factors (family and twin studies), sociocultural factors (feminine thinness is considered more attractive by many in western societies, leading to pressure to loss weight and to media stereotypes), occupational pressures, family environment (family relationships may exhibit enmeshment, overprotectiveness, rigidity and lack of conflict resolution; other family members may have an unusual interest in food), hypothalamic dysfunction, weight phobia.

Precipitating factors
There are usually no precipitating factors, but occasionally the onset may be associated with the occurrence of a stressful event.

Perpetuating factors
Sociocultural (as above), family environment (once started, the disorder may give the patient a central role in the family and may be perpetuated by its role in keeping the family together), individual (social withdrawal, weight checking, anxiety related to food and eating, difficulties coping with adolescence and adulthood).

Management

The condition should be explained to the patient and their family. The need for controlled weight gain should be agreed with the patient in the context of a therapeutic relationship.

Hospitalization
This is required if there is:

- Severe weight loss
- A high rate of weight loss
- Severe metabolic disturbance or infection
- A severe depressive episode or risk of suicide
- Failure to maintain the weight gain agreed in an outpatient contract
- A family crisis.

The admission should ideally be planned and mutually agreed, but if voluntary admission is refused and there is danger to life compulsory admission should be considered.

Inpatient treatment

This includes:

- Keeping *weight and fluid charts*
- *Controlled refeeding*
- A *behavioural regimen* may be used, e.g. starting with bed rest, which is gradually relaxed as weight is gained at a previously agreed rate
- *Psychotherapy*, initially supportive, but followed by cognitive and family therapies (see below) as progress is made.

Outpatient treatment

- *Supportive psychotherapy* helps to contain the difficulties encountered by the patient while she or he is aided in the process of keeping to an agreed diet, encouraged not to lose weight, and assisted in developing better interpersonal relationships.
- *Cognitive therapy* aims to identify and change inappropriate cognitions regarding eating behaviour, body weight, body shape, self-esteem and any tendency to perfectionism.
- *Family therapy* addresses features of the family environment that may play an aetiological role.

For both inpatients and outpatients other aspects of treatment may include the following.

Drug treatment

Antidepressants may be helpful, particularly if depressive, obsessional or anxiety symptoms exist. Chlorpromazine may be used to encourage weight gain.

Self-help groups

These may promote autonomy and provide mutual support. They are also helpful for relatives and may be a useful source of educational literature.

Educational material

Likewise, such material, including informative books, can be recommended to the patient and the family.

Prognosis

Early in the illness the course is often fluctuating, with alternate periods of remission and relapse. Medium-term outcome, 5–10 years after onset, is as follows:

- About 23% recover fully.
- In about 54% some degree of chronic or fluctuating psychiatric disturbance remains.
- About 23% remain severely ill.

Some patients go on to develop bulimia nervosa.

In the long term, over 20 years after onset, there is an 18% mortality, either directly from anorexia nervosa or from suicide. One factor that predicts a poor outcome is a long history of the illness at presentation.

BULIMIA NERVOSA
Clinical features

This is a syndrome characterized by repeated bouts of overeating and an excessive preoccupation with the control of body weight, with a morbid fear of fatness, leading the patient to adopt extreme measures so as to mitigate the 'fattening' effects of ingested food, e.g. through self-induced vomiting, purgative abuse and the abuse of appetite suppressants, thyroid preparations or diuretics (ICD-10). Patients often have a weight in the normal range and a normal menstrual cycle. A past history of anorexia nervosa is common but not invariable.

DSM-IV criteria for bulimia nervosa

These are:

- Recurrent episodes of binge-eating, which are characterized by both of the following:
  - Eating, in a discrete period of time (e.g. within any 2-hour period), an amount of food that is definitely larger than most people would eat during that same time and under similar circumstances
  - A sense of lack of control over eating during the episode

- Recurrent inappropriate compensatory behaviour in order to prevent weight gain, such as:
  - Self-induced vomiting
  - Misuse of laxatives
  - Misuse of diuretics
  - Misuse of ememas
  - Fasting
  - Excessive exercise
- The binge-eating and inappropriate compensatory behaviour both occur, on average, at least twice a week for 3 months
- Self-evaluation is unduly influenced by body shape and weight
- The disturbance does not occur exclusively during episodes of anorexia nervosa.

Purging type

During the current episode of bulimia nervosa the patient has regularly engaged in self-induced vomiting or the misuse of laxatives, diuretics or enemas.

Binge-eating/purging type

During the current episode of bulimia nervosa the patient has used other inappropriate compensatory behaviours, such as fasting or excessive exercise, but has not regularly engaged in self-induced vomiting or the misuse of laxatives, diuretics or enemas.

Physical examination and investigations

Repeated vomiting usually leads to disturbances of body electrolytes. Hypokalaemia is potentially fatal, and causes muscular weakness, cardiac arrhythmias and renal impairment. Other results of electrolyte disturbances include epileptic seizures, urinary tract infections and tetany. Enlargement of the salivary glands, particularly the parotids, may give the face a chubby appearance. Intermittent facial or peripheral oedema may also occur, particularly if purgatives are abused. The acidic gastric fluid leads to erosion of the enamel of the inner surfaces of the front teeth. If fingers are used to stimulate the gag reflex, calluses (Russell's sign) may form on the dorsum of the hand. Some of the complications of vomiting, purging and diuretic abuse are shown in Figure 8.2. The differential diagnosis of this disorder is summarized in Table 8.1.

Epidemiology

Point prevalence

In young women in the US and UK 1–2%; some estimates are up to 10%.

Age of onset

Usually in adolescence or early adult life.

Sex ratio

Rare in males.

Ethnicity

Rare in non-western countries.

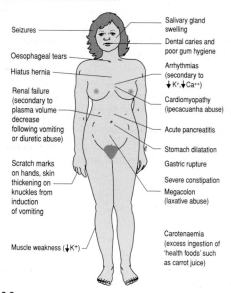

Figure 8.2
A typical cycle in bulimia nervosa. (After Garfinkel PF, Garner DM 1982 Anorexia nervosa: a multidimensional perspective, New York: Brunen Mazel. Reproduced with permission from Puri BK, Laking PJ, Treasaden IH 1996 Textbook of psychiatry. Edinburgh: Churchill Livingstone.)

Aetiology

Predisposing factors

A history of frank or subthreshold anorexia nervosa; a tendency to be overweight; predisposition to mood disorder and psychoactive substance abuse; borderline personality traits.

Perpetuating factors

Low self-esteem → excessive concern about body shape and weight → strict dieting → binge-eating → low self-esteem.

Management

Hospitalization

Although most cases can be managed as outpatients, hospitalization is indicated if there is:

- a severe depressive episode or risk of suicide
- poor physical health
- poor response to outpatient management
- first-trimester pregnancy (↑risk of spontaneous abortion).

Cognitive therapy

The patient is made responsible for controlling her own eating.

Drug treatment

Fluoxetine 60 mg/day (higher than the usual antidepressant dose).

Psychotherapies

Individual therapy, group psychotherapy and family work may be of help.

Self-help groups

These may promote autonomy and provide mutual support. They are also helpful for relatives and may be a useful source of educational literature.

Educational material

Likewise, such material, including informative books, can be recommended to the patient and the family.

Prognosis

There is a variable outcome; the disorder may last for many years.

Psychosexual and gender disorders

· ·

In this chapter the following psychosexual and gender disorders are outlined: sexual dysfunction (not secondary to organic disorder), gender identity disorders, and disorders of sexual preference.

· ·

SEXUAL RESPONSE
Normal anatomy

The normal anatomy of the female genitalia is shown in Figure 9.1, and that of the male genitalia in Figure 9.2. Patients with sexual dysfunction may not be aware of the structures shown, and therefore it is often helpful to show them such diagrams (or models).

Normal sexual response

In Masters and Johnson's model of the sexual response there are four phases (Figure 9.3).

Excitement phase
Arousal occurs in response to sexual stimulation (which may be fantasy as well as reality) and there is a desire to engage in sexual activity. In females the following occur during the excitement phase:

- A subjective sense of sexual pleasure
- Rapid vaginal lubrication
- Expansion and distension of the inner vagina
- Swelling and elongation of the clitoris
- Elevation of the uterus
- Nipple erection (in some women)
- Increased blood pressure
- Increased pulse.

Female external genitals

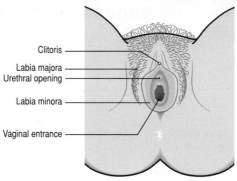

Clitoris
Labia majora
Urethral opening
Labia minora
Vaginal entrance

Female internal genitals

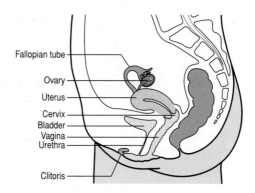

Fallopian tube
Ovary
Uterus
Cervix
Bladder
Vagina
Urethra
Clitoris

Figure 9.1
Female genitalia. (Reproduced with permission from Puri BK, Laking PJ,
Treasaden IH 1996 Textbook of psychiatry. Edinburgh: Churchill Livingstone.)

In males the following occur:

- Erection of the penis
- Thickening of the scrotal skin
- Elevation of the testes
- Increased blood pressure
- Increased pulse.

Male external genitals

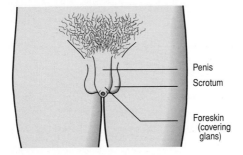

Penis

Scrotum

Foreskin
(covering
glans)

Male internal genitals

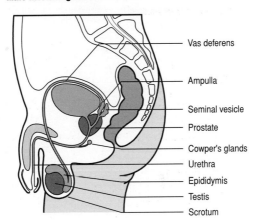

Vas deferens

Ampulla

Seminal vesicle

Prostate

Cowper's glands

Urethra

Epididymis

Testis

Scrotum

Figure 9.2
Male genitalia. (Reproduced with permission from Puri BK, Laking PJ, Treasaden IH 1996 Textbook of psychiatry. Edinburgh: Churchill Livingstone.)

Plateau phase

There is an intensification of the sexual excitement to a level from which orgasm can occur. In females the following occur:

- Breast enlargement
- Areolar enlargement

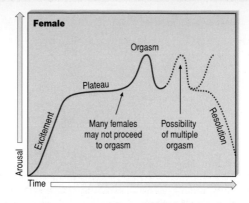

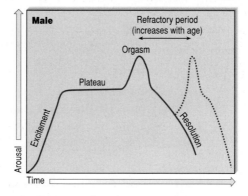

Figure 9.3
Relative timings of Masters and Johnson's phases of the sexual response. (Reproduced with permission from Puri BK, Laking PJ, Treasaden IH 1996 Textbook of psychiatry. Edinburgh: Churchill Livingstone.)

- Swelling of the outer third of the vagina
- Withdrawal of the clitoral head and shaft into the clitoral hood
- Reddening of the labia minora
- Increased muscle tension
- Increased blood pressure
- Increased pulse
- Occasionally a flush across the front of the trunk and head.

In males the following occur:

- Some change in colour in the head of the penis
- Enlargement of the testes
- Further elevation of the testes
- Increased muscle tension
- Increased blood pressure
- Increased pulse
- Occasionally a flush across the front of the trunk and head.

Orgasm phase

During this phase the sexual pleasure reaches a maximum, with an involuntary release of sexual tension and rhythmic contractions of the perineal muscles and reproductive organs. In females the following occur during orgasm:

- Rhythmic contractions of the outer third of the vagina – these are not always subjectively experienced by the woman
- Uterine contractions
- Rhythmic contractions of the anal sphincter
- Maximal pulse
- Maximal blood pressure
- Maximal respiratory rate.

In males the following occur during orgasm:

- The sensation of ejaculatory inevitability (during which ejaculation from the prostate and seminal vesicles and other glands contributes to the creation of seminal fluid), followed by rhythmic contractions of the urethra to cause ejaculation of the seminal fluid
- Rhythmic contractions of the anal sphincter
- Maximal pulse
- Maximal blood pressure
- Maximal respiratory rate.

Resolution phase

There is a sense of muscular relaxation and general well-being. In females the cervix is lowered to the vaginal floor and some gaping of the cervical os occurs. During this phase males are refractory to further penile erection and orgasm, whereas females are almost immediately able to achieve further orgasms.

SEXUAL DYSFUNCTION NOT CAUSED BY ORGANIC DISORDER OR DISEASE

Sexual dysfunction covers the various ways in which an individual is unable to participate in a sexual relationship as he or she would wish (ICD-10).

Organic causes of sexual dysfunction include physical disorders, the effects of medication, and excessive alcohol consumption. When a psychiatric disorder, such as a depressive episode, underlies the dysfunction then the diagnosis is of the psychiatric disorder itself.

Many types of non-organic sexual dysfunction share the following aetiological factors:

- Variable sexual drive between different people, possibly as a result of variable levels of sex hormones
- Ignorance of sexual matters
- Anxiety.

Lack or loss of sexual desire
Commoner in women. May be secondary to relationship difficulties or a depressive disorder.

Sexual aversion
The prospect of sexual interaction with a partner is associated with strong negative feelings and produces sufficient fear or anxiety that sexual activity is avoided (ICD-10).

Lack of sexual enjoyment
Sexual responses occur normally and orgasm is experienced but there is a lack of appropriate pleasure (ICD-10). It is commoner in women.

Failure of genital response
In men this manifests mainly as erectile dysfunction, in which there is difficulty in developing an erection or in maintaining it long enough for satisfactory sexual intercourse. If erection occurs normally in certain situations, for example on waking, during masturbation, or with other sexual partners, then the disorder is likely to be psychogenic rather than physiological in nature. It is commoner in older men. Erectile dysfunction may be secondary to low sexual drive, performance anxiety, reduced interest in the partner or a depressive episode.

In women it manifests mainly as vaginal dryness or failure of lubrication. Vaginal dryness may be a symptom of postmenopausal oestrogen deficiency.

Orgasmic dysfunction

Orgasm is markedly delayed or does not occur. If it is situational it is likely to be psychogenic rather than physiological in nature. It is commoner in women, in whom it may be the result of lack of foreplay, low sexual drive, lack of interest in the partner or tiredness.

Premature ejaculation

This is the regular occurrence of ejaculation before or too soon after vaginal penetration for the female partner to enjoy sexual intercourse. It is commoner in younger men, and often occurs in those with little or no previous experience of sexual intercourse.

Non-organic vaginismus

Vaginal muscle spasm occurs, occluding the vaginal opening and so making penetration impossible or painful. It may result from feelings of guilt.

Non-organic dyspareunia

This is non-organic pain occurring during sexual intercourse. It can occur in both women and men. In ICD-10 this category is used only if there is no other more primary sexual dysfunction, e.g. vaginismus.

Excessive sexual drive

In both sexes this is commoner during the late teenage years or early adulthood. It may be secondary to (hypo)mania or early dementia.

Assessment

In addition to a full history of the problem, a detailed history should also be taken of the level of sexual drive, sexual knowledge and technique, alcohol intake, and the relationship with the partner. The possibility that either partner is suffering from a psychiatric disorder (e.g. a depressive episode) should be examined. A physical examination and appropriate investigations should be carried out to exclude the possibility of an organic aetiology. Common organic causes of erectile dysfunction are given in Table 9.1.

Table 9.1 Organic causes of erectile dysfunction. (After Zongheim J. Diagnosis and management of endocrine disorders of erectile dysfunction. *Urological Clinics of North America* 1995; 22:789–802)

Diabetes mellitus	40%
Vascular disease	30%
Radical surgery	13%
Spinal cord injury	8%
Endocrine disorders	6%
Multiple sclerosis	3%

Management

Sex therapy

Masters and Johnson are largely responsible for sex therapy, which consists of the following:

- *Both partners are treated together*.
- *Education:* the patient and their partner may need education about the anatomical, physiological and emotional aspects of sexual intercourse and sexual responses.
- *Communication:* both partners should be encouraged to be open with each other about their sexual wishes and what they find enjoyable during foreplay and intercourse.
- *Graded sexual tasks:* initially both partners are encouraged to touch and caress each other anywhere except the genital areas (sensate focus stage). In the next stage they are encouraged to give pleasure without engaging in intercourse; communication with the partner is relied on and mutual masturbation allowed. Finally, full sexual intercourse is permitted.

Pharmacological treatments

Pharmacological treatments for erectile dysfunction should be used with caution if the penis is deformed, for example in the following conditions:

- Angulation
- Cavernosal fibrosis
- Peyronie's disease.

Drugs that may be used to treat erectile dysfunction (after excluding treatable organic causes) include:

- *Alprostadil (prostaglandin E₁)* is administered by intracavernosal injection or intraurethral application; it may also be used as a diagnostic test. Important side effects include penile pain and priapism, as well as reactions at the injection site.
- *Sildenafil (Viagra)* is an orally administered phosphodiesterase inhibitor that enhances the action of nitric oxide on smooth muscle and increases penile blood flow. Important side effects include dyspepsia, headache, flushing, dizziness, visual disturbances, nasal congestion and priapism. It should not be administered to those receiving nitrates. Other contraindications include recent stroke, recent myocardial infarction, a blood pressure below 90/50 (systolic and diastolic, measured in mmHg), and hereditary degenerative retinal disorders.

Special techniques
Vaginal dilators of gradually increasing size can be used in cases of vaginismus. For premature ejaculation the squeeze technique or stop–start method can be used. For erectile dysfunction vacuum devices may be used to achieve an erection, which may then be maintained for sexual intercourse by slipping a device such as a tight rubber band or plastic annulus over the base of the penis.

Marital (couple) therapy
This is indicated when conflict in the relationship is the underlying cause of the sexual dysfunction.

GENDER IDENTITY DISORDERS
Transsexualism

A desire to live and be accepted as a member of the opposite sex, usually accompanied by a sense of discomfort with one's anatomical sex and a wish to have treatment (hormonal and surgical) to make one's body as congruent as possible with the preferred sex (ICD-10). Psychotherapy is offered initially. In a few specialist centres gender reassignment surgery is offered only after extensive discussion, planning and preparation, during which the person lives as if of the opposite sex for a long period; during this time hormonal treatment may be administered.

Dual-role transvestism

In this disorder the individual occasionally wears clothes of the opposite sex (cross-dressing) but does not wish to become a member of that sex. The cross-dressing is not accompanied by sexual excitement.

Gender identity disorder of childhood

A pervasive and persistent desire, present well before puberty, to be, or to insist that one is, of the opposite sex.

DISORDERS OF SEXUAL PREFERENCE

In these disorders, also called **paraphilias**, sexual arousal occurs in response to objects or situations that are not normal arousal stimuli and which may interfere with affectionate reciprocal sexual acts. Table 9.2 lists several types of paraphilia, together with the corresponding arousing stimuli, about which there are recurrent intense sexual urges and sexually arousing fantasies.

Table 9.2 Disorders of sexual preference

Disorder	Arousing stimulus
Fetishism	Non-living object (fetish), e.g. rubber, plastic or leather objects
Fetishistic transvestism	Wearing clothes of the opposite sex
Exhibitionism	Exposure of one's genitals to a stranger
Voyeurism	Observing unsuspecting people undressing and/or engaging in sexual or intimate behaviour (unlike in pornography, where those being observed know they are being seen)
Paedophilia	Sexual activity with a prepubescent child
Sadomasochism	Sexual activity involving bondage or the infliction of pain or humiliation (a masochist prefers to be the recipient of such stimulation, whereas a sadist prefers to be its provider)
Frotteurism	Touching and rubbing against a non-consenting person
Necrophilia	Sexual activity with a corpse
Zoophilia	Animals are incorporated into sexual arousal fantasies and sexual activity, including masturbation, orogenital interactions and intercourse
Coprophilia	Sexual pleasure is associated with passing faeces on to the partner or being defecated upon by the partner
Klismaphilia	Sexual pleasure is associated with the insertion of an enema per rectum
Urophilia	Sexual pleasure is associated with passing urine on to the partner or being urinated upon by the partner

Personality disorders

Personality disorders are defined in ICD-10 as deeply ingrained and enduring behaviour patterns manifesting as inflexible responses to a broad range of personal and social situations. They represent extreme or significant deviations from the way average individuals in a given culture perceive, think, feel and relate to others. They are often associated with subjective distress and problems in social functioning and performance. They tend to appear in late childhood or adolescence and continue to be manifest into adulthood; it is therefore unlikely that a diagnosis of personality disorder is appropriate in those under the age of 17.

TYPES

Paranoid personality disorder

There is a tendency to interpret the actions of others as being deliberately demeaning or threatening. An excessive sensitivity to setbacks occurs and there is a tendency to bear grudges, to be suspicious, and to be preoccupied with unsubstantiated conspiratorial explanations of events.

Schizoid personality disorder

There is an indifference to social relationships and a restricted range of emotional experience and expression. Few, if any, activities give pleasure and individuals tend to be emotionally cold, detached or flat, with a limited ability to express feelings of warmth or anger towards others. Solitary activities are preferred and there is a preoccupation with fantasy and introspection.

Dissocial (antisocial) personality disorder

Irresponsible and antisocial behaviour takes place, manifested by a callous unconcern for others, a disregard for social norms and obligations, incapacity to maintain (though not to establish) enduring relationships, a low threshold for frustration and anger, and an incapacity to feel guilt or learn from being punished.

Emotionally unstable personality disorder

There is a tendency to act impulsively without considering the consequences, together with affective instability. Two types of emotionally unstable personality disorder can be distinguished:

- *Impulsive:* there is emotional instability, lack of impulse control, and often violent outbursts in response to criticism
- *Borderline:* there is emotional instability, and disturbance of self-image, long-term goals and internal preference, which may lead to chronic feelings of emptiness, unstable interpersonal relationships and impulsive actions (e.g. shopping sprees, shoplifting and casual sexual relationships).

Histrionic personality disorder

There is excessive emotionality and attention-seeking, with self-dramatization, theatricality, suggestibility, shallow and labile affectivity, and overconcern with physical attractiveness. Excitement is continually sought, as is the appreciation of others and activities that allow one to be the centre of attention.

Anankastic (obsessive–compulsive) personality disorder

There is a tendency to perfectionism and inflexibility. There may be a preoccupation with rules and regulations and an unreasonable insistence that others do things the same way. Decision making is avoided or postponed. Unwelcome thoughts or impulses may continually intrude.

Anxious (avoidant) personality disorder

There is a tendency to social discomfort, a fear of being thought of in a negative way, and timidity. There may be a belief that one is socially inept and inferior, and an avoidance of activities and involvement with others owing to a fear of criticism or rejection.

Dependent personality disorder

There is a tendency towards dependent and submissive behaviour, in which others are encouraged or allowed to make one's important decisions and one is unwilling to make any demands on people one depends on. Being alone feels uncomfortable owing to feelings of helplessness. There is difficulty in initiating projects.

MANAGEMENT

In the assessment of the patient interviewing independent informants is very important. Organic causes need to be excluded, e.g. cerebral disorder and epilepsy. Any additional psychiatric disorder should be identified. In making a diagnosis of a personality disorder it is important to establish that it has been present since adolescence. Therapeutic strategies that may be helpful include supervision and support, group therapy and the therapeutic community.

Child and adolescent psychiatry

The disorders outlined in this chapter are ones that usually appear during childhood or adolescence.

CHILDHOOD DEVELOPMENT

Normal childhood development is summarized in Table 11.1.

CHILD PSYCHIATRIC INTERVIEW

The assessment of a child requires the gathering of information from all relevant sources, such as the child's family, teachers, doctor, social workers, paediatricians and the police (in the case of conduct problems, for example). More than one assessment interview may be required, and the family is usually asked to attend. (However, in the case of suspected child abuse the child should be interviewed without the presence of the suspected abuser.) Table 11.2 summarizes the information to be gathered at such an interview.

PREVALENCE OF PSYCHIATRIC DISORDER

A study by Rutter and colleagues of 10- and 11-year-olds in the Isle of Wight in 1970 found that the 1-year prevalence of psychiatric disorder was 6.8%, with the rate in boys being twice that in girls. Of the 6.8%, 3% had conduct disorder and 2% emotional disorder. The prevalence increased with reduced IQ, and there was a strong association with physical handicap and particularly with brain injury. A similar survey in an inner London borough, in which there was a high prevalence of overcrowding, found that the 1-year prevalence of psychiatric disorder was 13%, double that in the Isle of Wight.

Table 11.1 Childhood development and developmental stages (Reproduced with permission from Puri BK, Laking PJ, Treasaden IH 1996 Textbook of psychiatry. Edinburgh: Churchill Livingstone.)

Age	Milestones	Freudian stage	Piagetian stage	Ericksonian stage
0–6 months	Vocalizes up to double-syllable sounds, rolls over, objects — palmar grasp, hand to hand and to mouth, smiles and laughs	Oral	Sensorimotor	Trust vs. mistrust
6 months to 1 year	Crawls, stands with support, sits unsupported, pincer grasp present, stranger shyness	Oral	Sensorimotor	Trust vs. mistrust
1–2 years	Walks, runs, builds up to 2–3 word sentences, feeds self with spoon, parallel play, beginning to attain continence	Anal	Sensorimotor	Autonomy vs. shame and doubt
3–5 years	Attains continence, cooperative play, draws a man, much questioning, speech increases in fluency, learns to skip and hop and to dress and undress	Phallic	Preoperational	Initiative vs. guilt
6 years to puberty (middle childhood)	Increasing involvement with peer group, schooling, increased autonomy	Latency	Concrete operational	Industry vs. inferiority
Adolescence	Moves towards independence, relates mostly to peer group	Genital	Formal operational	Identity vs. confusion

Table 11.2 Information to be amassed in a child psychiatric interview (Reproduced with permission from Eminson M, Chapter 6 in D Black, D Cottrell (eds) 1993 Seminars in child and adolescent psychiatry. London: Gaskell.)

Source and nature of referral
- Who made referral?
- Who initiated referral?
- Family attitudes to referral

Description of presenting complaints
- Onset, frequency, intensity, duration, location (home, school etc.)
- Antecedents and consequences
- Ameliorating and exacerbating factors
- Specific examples
- Parental and family beliefs about causation
- Past attempts to solve problem

Description of child's current general functioning
- School
    behaviour and emotions
    academic performance
    peer and staff relationships
- Peer relationships generally
- Family relationships

Personal/developmental history
- Pregnancy, labour, delivery
- Early developmental milestones
- Separations/disruptions
- Physical illnesses and their meaning for parents
- Reactions to school
- Puberty
- Temperamental style

Family history
- Personal and social histories of both parents especially
    history of mental illness
    their experience of being parented
- History of family development
    how parents came together
    history of pregnancies
    separations and effects on children
- Who lives at home currently
- Strengths/weaknesses of all at home
- Current social stresses and supports

Information from observation of family interaction:
structure, organization, communication, sensitivity

Information from observation of child at interview:
motor, sensory, speech, language, social relating skills

Mental state, concerns, and spontaneous account if age appropriate

Results of physical examination

Plan for future investigation and management

HYPERKINETIC DISORDER OR ATTENTION-DEFICIT/HYPERACTIVITY DISORDER (ADHD)

The cluster of age-inappropriate behavioural abnormalities of the triad

- Inattention
- Hyperactivity
- Impulsivity

constitutes the core of the ICD-10 diagnostic group of disorders known as hyperkinetic disorder, and known in DSM-IV as attention-deficit/hyperactivity disorder (often abbreviated to ADHD). The first two abnormalities are particularly important for the ICD-10 diagnosis. The clinical features in the next subsection are mainly based on the ICD-10 criteria; those of DSM-IV follow after it. Although ADHD is considered in this chapter on children and adolescents, it should be borne in mind that it can also occur in adults.

Clinical features

There is impaired attention and overactivity, and both occur in more than one situation, e.g. at home, in school, at a clinic. Impaired attention leads to frequent changes from one activity to another, and to unfinished activities. Overactivity manifests as excessive restlessness, e.g. running and jumping around, noisiness and excessive talkativeness.

Associated features include disinhibition in social relationships, recklessness and the impulsive defying of rules.

For an ICD-10 diagnosis these behaviour problems should start before the age of 6 years and be of long duration.

DSM-IV criteria for attention-deficit/ hyperactivity disorder

A. Either (1) or (2):

(1) At least six of the following symptoms of **inattention** have persisted for at least 6 months to a degree that is maladaptive and inconsistent with developmental level:

(a) often fails to give close attention to details or makes careless mistakes in schoolwork, work or other activities

(b) often has difficulty sustaining attention in tasks or play activities

(c) often does not seem to listen when spoken to directly

(d) often does not follow through on instructions and fails to finish schoolwork, chores, or duties in the workplace (not because of difficulty understanding instructions)

(e) often has difficulty organizing tasks and activities

(f) often avoids, dislikes or is reluctant to engage in tasks that require sustained mental effort (e.g. schoolwork or homework)

(g) often loses things necessary for tasks and activities

(h) is often easily distracted by extraneous stimuli

(i) is often forgetful in daily activities.

(2) At least six of the following symptoms of **hyperactivity** (a–f) – **impulsivity** (g–i) have persisted for at least 6 months to a degree that is maladaptive and inconsistent with developmental level:

(a) often fidgets with hands or feet or squirms in seat

(b) often leaves seat in classroom or in other situations in which remaining seated is expected

(c) often runs about or climbs excessively in situations in which it is inappropriate (in adolescents and adults may be limited to subjective feelings of restlessness)

(d) often has difficulty playing or engaging in leisure activities quietly

(e) is often 'on the go', or often acts as if 'driven by a motor'

(f) often talks excessively

(g) often blurts out answers before questions have been completed

(h) often has difficulty awaiting turn

(i) often interrupts or intrudes on others (e.g. butts into conversations or games).

B. Some hyperactive–impulsive or inattentive symptoms that caused impairment were present before the age of 7 years.

C. Some impairment from the symptoms is present in two or more settings (e.g. at school/work and at home).

D. There must be clear evidence of clinically significant impairment in social, academic or occupational functioning.

E. The symptoms do not occur exclusively during a pervasive developmental disorder (e.g. autism, Rett's disorder, Asperger's disorder), schizophrenia or other psychotic disorder, and are not better accounted for by another mental disorder (e.g. mood disorder, anxiety disorder, dissociative disorder or a personality disorder).

Epidemiology

Prevalence

In the UK hyperkinetic disorders have been found to have a prevalence of up to 20–30 per 1000 children. The prevalence of attention-deficit/hyperactivity disorder in the US is around 30–50 per 1000 in school-age children. This much higher prevalence in America may be partly the result of differences in diagnosis or terminology.

Social class

Hyperkinetic disorders are commoner in those living in poor social conditions.

Sex ratio

This disorder is much more common in males. Male:female ratio ranges from 4:1 to 9:1.

Aetiology

Genetic (studies of adopted children), biochemical and social factors have been suggested.

Management

Support and advice

For parents and teachers.

Remedial teaching
Behaviour modification
Appropriate methods can be taught to parents and teachers to prevent reinforcement of the problem behaviour.

Drug treatment
Under specialist supervision CNS stimulants (e.g. methylphenidate, pemoline) can be used. Such use must be selective because of the side-effects, such as irritability, depressed mood, insomnia, reduced appetite and retarded growth.

Prognosis

The symptoms often cease by puberty, although in severe cases they may continue into adult life.

....

CONDUCT DISORDER
Clinical features

The characteristic features are a repetitive and persistent pattern of dissocial, aggressive or defiant conduct, which at its most extreme amounts to major violations of age-appropriate social expectations and is therefore more severe than ordinary childish mischief or adolescent rebelliousness (ICD-10). An isolated dissocial or criminal act is not sufficient to make this diagnosis, for which an enduring pattern of dissocial behaviour is required.

DSM-IV criteria for conduct disorder

A. A repetitive and persistent pattern of behaviour in which the basic rights of others or major age-appropriate societal norms or rules are violated, as manifested by the presence of at least three of the following criteria in the past 12 months, with at least one criterion present in the past 6 months:

Aggression to people and animals

(1) Often bullies, threatens, or intimidates others
(2) Often initiates physical fights

(3) Has used a weapon that can cause serious physical harm to others
(4) Has been physically cruel to people
(5) Has been physically cruel to animals
(6) Has stolen while confronting a victim (e.g. mugging, purse snatching, extortion, armed robbery)
(7) Has forced someone into sexual activity

Destruction of property
(8) Has deliberately engaged in fire setting with the intention of causing serious damage
(9) Has deliberately destroyed others' property (other than by fire setting)

Deceitfulness or theft
(10) Has broken into someone else's house, building or car
(11) Often lies to obtain goods or favours or to avoid obligations (i.e. 'cons' others)
(12) Has stolen items of non-trivial value without confronting a victim (e.g. shoplifting, but without breaking and entering; forgery)

Serious violations of rules
(13) Often stays out at night despite parental prohibitions, beginning before the age of 13 years
(14) Has run away from home overnight at least twice while living in parental or parental surrogate home (or once without returning for a lengthy period)
(15) Is often truant from school, beginning before the age of 13 years.

B. The disturbance in behaviour causes clinically significant impairment in social, academic or occupational functioning.
C. If the individual is aged 18 the criteria are not met for antisocial personality disorder.

Epidemiology

Prevalence

In the Isle of Wight study the prevalence was found to be 3%; in an inner London borough it was double this.

Sex ratio

Commoner in boys.

Aetiology

Social factors (commoner in those from deprived areas, broken homes, and those who have been in residential care in early childhood), genetic factors (adoption studies) and brain damage have been suggested. Aetiological factors are summarized in Figure 11.1.

Management

In severe cases social case-work, family therapy, behaviour therapy and group therapy may be required. Milder cases

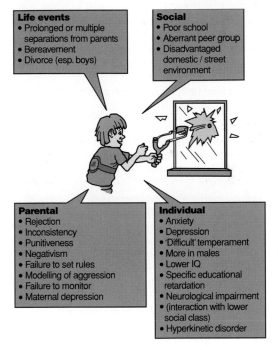

Life events
- Prolonged or multiple separations from parents
- Bereavement
- Divorce (esp. boys)

Social
- Poor school
- Aberrant peer group
- Disadvantaged domestic / street environment

Parental
- Rejection
- Inconsistency
- Punitiveness
- Negativism
- Failure to set rules
- Modelling of aggression
- Failure to monitor
- Maternal depression

Individual
- Anxiety
- Depression
- 'Difficult' temperament
- More in males
- Lower IQ
- Specific educational retardation
- Neurological impairment
- (interaction with lower social class)
- Hyperkinetic disorder

Figure 11.1
Aetiological factors in conduct disorder. (Reproduced with permission from Puri BK, Laking PJ, Treasaden IH 1996 Textbook of psychiatry. Edinburgh: Churchill Livingstone.)

may abate without such treatment, with counselling and practical support being offered to the parents.

Prognosis

Two-thirds continue to have problems in adult life. Poor prognostic factors include:

- Many and varied symptoms
- Problems at home
- Problems in the community
- Anti-authoritarian and aggressive attitudes.

....

(S)ELECTIVE MUTISM
Clinical features

There is characteristically a marked, emotionally determined selectivity in speaking, such that the child demonstrates language competence in some situations but fails to speak in other (definable) situations (ICD-10).

DSM-IV criteria for selective mutism

A. Consistent failure to speak in specific social situations (in which there is an expectation for speaking, e.g. at school) despite speaking in other situations.
B. The disturbance interferes with educational or occupational achievement, or with social communication.
C. The duration of the disturbance is at least 1 month (not limited to the first month of school).
D. The failure to speak is not caused by a lack of knowledge of, or comfort with, the spoken language required in the social situation.
E. The disturbance is not better accounted for by a communication disorder (e.g. stuttering) and does not occur exclusively during the course of a pervasive developmental disorder, schizophrenia or other psychotic disorder.

Epidemiology
Prevalence
About 1 per 1000 children.

Age of onset
Usually first manifests in early childhood.

Sex ratio
Equal.

Management

Psychotherapy, family therapy behaviour modification and speech therapy have been used.

Prognosis

Fifty per cent have a good prognosis. A poor prognosis is indicated by a failure to improve by the age of 10 years.

....

STUTTERING (STAMMERING)
Clinical features

The speech is characterized by frequent repetition or prolongation of syllables or words, or by frequent hesitations leading to a disruption in rhythm and fluency. It occurs normally and transiently at 3–4 years of age.

DSM-IV criteria for stuttering

A. Disturbance in the normal fluency and time patterning of speech (inappropriate for the individual's age), characterized by frequent occurrences of one or more of the following:

(1) Sound and syllable repetitions
(2) Sound prolongations
(3) Interjections
(4) Broken words (e.g. pauses within a word)
(5) Audible or silent blocking (filled or unfilled pauses in speech)
(6) Circumlocutions (word substitutions to avoid problematic words)
(7) Words produced with an excess of physical tension
(8) Monosyllabic whole-word repetitions (e.g. 'I-I-I-I see him').

B. The disturbance in fluency interferes with academic or occupational achievement, or with social communication.

C. If a speech–motor or sensory deficit is present, the speech difficulties are in excess of those usually associated with these problems.

Epidemiology

Prevalence

About 1% in prepubertal children, dropping to 0.8% in adolescence.

Sex ratio

Male:female = 3:1–4:1.

Aetiology

There is evidence of a genetic factor (from family and twin studies).

Management

No effective treatment exists; speech therapy is often tried.

Prognosis

It persists in about 3% of the general population.

··
FUNCTIONAL (NON–ORGANIC) ENURESIS
Clinical features

This is the involuntary passage of urine, by day and/or by night, which is abnormal in relation to the individual's mental age and which is not the result of a physical disorder. Normal bladder control usually occurs by the age of 5 years. Enuresis present from birth is called primary; that arising after a period of acquired bladder control is called secondary.

DSM-IV criteria for enuresis

A. Repeated voiding of urine into bed or clothes (whether involuntary or intentional).

B. The behaviour is clinically significant as manifested by either a frequency of twice a week for at least 3 consecutive months, or the presence of clinically significant distress or impairment in social, academic (occupational) or other important areas of functioning.
C. Chronological age is at least 5 years (or equivalent developmental level).
D. The behaviour is not caused exclusively by the direct physiological effect of a substance (e.g. a diuretic) or a general medical condition (e.g. diabetes, spina bifida, seizure disorder).

Epidemiology
Prevalence
About 10% of 5-year-olds, 5% of 10-year-olds and 1% of 15-year-olds, for nocturnal enuresis (bedwetting). The prevalence of diurnal (daytime) enuresis is lower.

Sex ratio
Nocturnal enuresis is commoner in boys, and diurnal enuresis in girls.

Aetiology
Genetic factors (family and twin studies), psychiatric disorder, recent life events and social disadvantage are possible causes. These are summarized in Figure 11.2.

Management
Assessment
Exclude physical causes, including urinary tract infection, diabetes mellitus, epilepsy, other neurological disorder, and structural abnormality of the urinary tract. Psychiatric causes should also be excluded.

Fluid intake
In the case of functional nocturnal enuresis parents should be advised to limit the child's intake of fluid before bedtime.

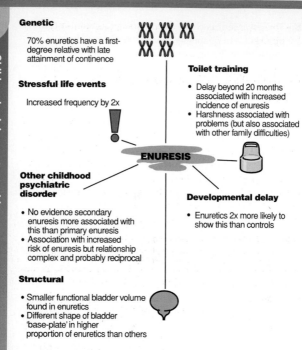

Genetic

70% enuretics have a first-degree relative with late attainment of continence

Stressful life events

Increased frequency by 2x

Toilet training

- Delay beyond 20 months associated with increased incidence of enuresis
- Harshness associated with problems (but also associated with other family difficulties)

ENURESIS

Other childhood psychiatric disorder

- No evidence secondary enuresis more associated with this than primary enuresis
- Association with increased risk of enuresis but relationship complex and probably reciprocal

Developmental delay

- Enuretics 2x more likely to show this than controls

Structural

- Smaller functional bladder volume found in enuretics
- Different shape of bladder 'base-plate' in higher proportion of enuretics than others

Figure 11.2
Aetiology of functional enuresis. (Reproduced with permission from Puri BK, Laking PJ, Treasaden IH 1996 Textbook of psychiatry. Edinburgh: Churchill Livingstone.)

Star chart
The child can be rewarded with stars on a chart for keeping dry.

Bell-and-pad
If the above measures do not help a buzzer or bell-and-pad method, in which a bell sounds when urine is passed and wets a pad under the sheets, is used. This can be combined with the star chart method.

Drug treatment
A small dose of a tricyclic antidepressant will usually stop enuresis, owing to its antimuscarinic action. However, disadvantages include a high relapse rate, side effects and

the toxicity risk in accidental or intentional overdose (e.g. by siblings).

FUNCTIONAL (NON-ORGANIC) ENCOPRESIS
Clinical features

This is the repeated voluntary or involuntary passage of faeces, usually of normal or near-normal consistency, in inappropriate places after an age at which bowel control is usual, in the absence of an organic cause. Encopresis present from birth is called primary; that arising after a period of acquired bowel control is called secondary. Table 11.3 summarizes the presentation of encopresis.

Table 11.3 Presentation of faecal soiling (encopresis) (Reproduced with permission from Puri BK, Laking PJ, Treasaden IH 1996 Textbook of psychiatry. Edinburgh: Churchill Livingstone.)

Consistency of faeces	Normal, loose or constipated
Place deposited	In pants, hidden or in 'significant' places (e.g. in a particular person's cupboard)
Development	Never continent (continuous), after period of continence (discontinuous) or regression (in various contexts — see below)
Activity	Smearing, anal fingering, or masturbation
Context	Power battle, upsetting life events (e.g. sexual abuse, divorce) and/or other psychiatric disorder
Physical	With soreness, anal fissures etc., or with normal anus

DSM-IV criteria for encopresis

A. Repeated passage of faeces into inappropriate places (e.g. clothing or the floor), whether involuntary or intentional.
B. At least one such event a month for at least 3 months.
C. Chronological age is at least 4 years (or equivalent developmental level).
D. The behaviour is not caused exclusively by the direct physiological effects of a substance (e.g. a laxative) or a

general medical condition, except through a mechanism involving constipation.

Epidemiology

Prevalence

Incontinent of faeces at least once per week occurs in 6% of 3-year-olds and 1.5% of 7-year-olds.

Sex ratio

Boys:girls = 3:1–4:1.

Aetiology

The aetiology of encopresis is summarized in Table 11.4.

Table 11.4 Aetiology of encopresis (Reproduced with permission from Puri BK, Laking PJ, Treasaden IH 1996 Textbook of psychiatry. Edinburgh: Churchill Livingstone)

Congenital	Constitutional variability can include bowel control
Individual	Developmental delay Physical trigger — anal fissure — constipation (low-roughage diet) — other bowel disorders
Parent – child	Coercive toilet training Emotional abuse or neglect 'Battleground' for relationship problems
Wider environment	Sexual abuse Family disharmony

Management

Assessment

Exclude physical causes such as chronic constipation. Assess emotional factors.

Behavioural

A programme in which the child is rewarded (e.g. star chart) for successfully passing faeces following each meal may prove successful.

Psychotherapy

Individual psychotherapy and family therapy may be required if there are emotional difficulties and/or problems with the relationship between the child and parent(s).

Drug treatment

Microenemata, smooth muscle stimulants, stool softeners, bulk agents and suppositories may be variously required (e.g. in retention).

Prognosis

Usually resolves by adolescence.

....
PICA
Clinical features

This is the persistent eating of substances normally considered inedible, e.g. soil, paint chippings and paper.

DSM-IV criteria for pica

A. Persistent eating of non-nutritive substances for at least 1 month.
B. The eating of non-nutritive substances is inappropriate to the developmental level.
C. The eating behaviour is not part of a culturally sanctioned practice.
D. If the eating behaviour occurs exclusively during the course of another mental disorder (e.g. mental retardation, pervasive developmental disorder, schizophrenia), it is sufficiently severe to warrant independent clinical attention.

Management

Brain damage and learning disabilities (mental retardation) should be excluded. The child should be kept away from the inedible substance(s).

Prognosis

Usually resolves as the child grows older.

TIC DISORDERS
Clinical features

There is some form of tic, that is, a rapid involuntary recurrent non-rhythmic motor movement, or vocal production, of sudden onset and with no apparent purpose. In Gilles de la Tourette syndrome complex tics, involving the limbs and trunk, occur together with echolalia, echopraxia, coprolalia (uttering obscenities) and copropraxia (making obscene gestures).

DSM-IV criteria for Tourette's disorder

A. Both multiple motor and one or more vocal tics have been present at some time during the illness, although not necessarily concurrently. (A **tic** is a sudden, rapid, recurrent, non-rhythmic stereotyped motor movement or vocalization.)

B. The tics occur many times a day (usually in bouts) nearly every day or intermittently throughout a period of more than 1 year, and during this period there is never a tic-free period of more than 3 consecutive months.

C. The disturbance causes marked distress or significant impairment in social, occupational or other important areas of functioning.

D. The onset is before the age of 18 years.

E. The disturbance is not caused by the direct physiological effects of a substance (e.g. stimulants) or a general medical condition (e.g. Huntington's disease or postviral encephalitis).

DSM-IV criteria for chronic motor or vocal tic disorder

A. Single or multiple motor or vocal tics, but not both, have been present at some time during the illness.

B. The tics occur many times a day nearly every day or intermittently throughout a period of more than 1 year, and during this period there was never a tic-free period of more than 3 consecutive months.

C. The disturbance causes marked distress or significant impairment in social, occupational or other important areas of functioning.
D. The onset is before the age of 18 years.
E. The disturbance is not caused by the direct physiological effects of a substance (e.g. stimulants) or a general medical condition (e.g. Huntington's disease or postviral encephalitis).
F. Criteria for Tourette's disorder have never been met.

DSM-IV criteria for transient tic disorder

A. Single or multiple motor and/or vocal tics.
B. The tics occur many times a day nearly every day for at least 4 weeks, but for no longer than 12 consecutive months.
C. The disturbance causes marked distress or significant impairment in social, occupational, or other important areas of functioning.
D. The onset is before the age of 18 years.
E. The disturbance is not caused by the direct physiological effects of a substance (e.g. stimulants) or a general medical condition (e.g. Huntington's disease or postviral encephalitis).
F. Criteria have never been met for Tourette's disorder or chronic motor or vocal tic disorder.

Epidemiology

Prevalence

Ten to 20% of children show transient tics at some time. Gilles de la Tourette syndrome is rare, occurring in approximately 4–5 individuals per 10 000, and can occur in adults as well as in children and adolescents.

Sex ratio

Commoner in males. For Gilles de la Tourette syndrome, male:female ratio is approximately 1.5:1–3:1.

Aetiology

Causes of tics are summarized in Table 11.5.

Table 11.5 Aetiology of tics (Reproduced with permission from Puri BK, Laking PJ, Treasaden IH 1996 Textbook of psychiatry. Edinburgh: Churchill Livingstone.)

Family	Family clusters reported, especially Tourette's
	Prevalence of multiple tics in 14–24% of first-degree relatives of patients with Tourette's
	Increased family psychopathology in families of ticqueurs although may be cause or effect
Individual	No gross neurological abnormalities
	Increased incidence of 'soft' neurological signs and 'non-specific' EEG changes
	Some verbal – performance discrepancies in functioning
	Some neuroleptic medications effective in controlling tics
	Tics exacerbated by dopamine agonists
	Wide range of psychological mechanisms proposed for tic disorders, from the psychoanalytic to the classically behavioural
	Tic movements have been shown to mimic involuntary startle responses to sudden stimulus

Management

Education

Education, advice and reassurance for the child and parents may be all that is required for simple tics.

Behavioural

Relaxation or massed practice may help.

Medication

In severe cases, e.g. Gilles de la Tourette syndrome, the antipsychotics haloperidol or pimozide may be useful.

ASPERGER'S SYNDROME

Clinical features

This is a disorder characterized by the same kind of abnormalities of social interaction that occur in autism, together with a restricted, stereotyped, repetitive repertoire of interests and activities, but which differs from autism primarily in that there is no general delay or retardation in language or in cognitive development (ICD-10). Psychotic episodes may occur in early adult life.

DSM-IV criteria for Asperger's disorder

A. Qualitative impairment in social interaction, as manifested by at least two of the following:

   (1) Marked impairment in the use of multiple non-verbal behaviours, such as eye-to-eye gaze, facial expression, body postures, and gestures to regulate social interaction
   (2) Failure to develop peer relationships appropriate to developmental level
   (3) A lack of spontaneous seeking to share enjoyment, interests or achievements with others (e.g. by a lack of showing, bringing or pointing out objects of interest to other people)
   (4) Lack of social or emotional reciprocity.

B. Restricted repetitive and stereotyped patterns of behaviour, interests and activities, as manifested by at least one of the following:

   (1) Encompassing preoccupation with one or more stereotyped and restricted patterns of interest that is abnormal either in intensity or focus
   (2) Apparently inflexible adherence to specific non-functional routines or rituals
   (3) Stereotyped and repetitive motor mannerisms (e.g. hand or finger flapping or twisting, or complex whole-body movements)
   (4) Persistent preoccupation with parts of objects.

C. The disturbance causes clinically significant impairment in social, occupational or other important areas of functioning.

D. There is no clinically significant general delay in language.

E. There is no clinically significant delay in cognitive development or in the development of age-appropriate self-help skills, adaptive behaviour (other than in social interaction) and curiosity about the environment in childhood.

F. Criteria are not met for another specific pervasive developmental disorder or for schizophrenia.

Epidemiology

Sex ratio
Boys:girls = 6:1–8:1.

Aetiology

This is unknown.

Prognosis

There is a strong tendency for the abnormalities to persist into adult life. Most can work, but few develop successful relationships with others.

12 People with learning disability (mental retardation)

ICD-10 defines mental retardation as a condition of arrested or incomplete development of the mind, which is especially characterized by impairment of skills manifested during the developmental period which contribute to the overall level of intelligence, i.e. cognitive, language, motor and social abilities. Retardation can occur with or without any other mental or physical disorder.

Those with this condition are also known variously as people with learning disability (or disabilities), people with learning difficulties, or, particularly in the past in the UK, as having a mental handicap.

CLASSIFICATION

The intelligence quotient is calculated from the following formula:

$$IQ = [(\text{mental age})/(\text{chronological age})].100$$

On the basis of IQ, ICD-10 classifies mental retardation into the groups shown in Table 12.1.

Table 12.1 Classification of mental retardation by IQ

Degree of mental retardation	IQ range
Mild	50–69 (inclusive)
Moderate	35–49 (inclusive)
Severe	20–34 (inclusive)
Profound	under 20

PREVALENCE

The overall prevalence of mental retardation is around 2%. Table 12.2 shows the prevalence of each type and Table 12.3 (page 182) shows the proportion.

Table 12.2 Prevalence of mental retardation

Degree of mental retardation	Prevalence (%)
Mild	1.5
Moderate and severe	0.5
Profound	0.05

Although IQ is standardized to follow a normal distribution, with mean 100 and standard deviation 15, the actual frequency distribution of IQ in the population is skewed in the way shown in Figure 12.1. The 'excess cases' with low IQ (over and above those expected on the grounds of probability to fall into that range of intelligence quotients) contain subjects with genetic and chromosomal abnormalities.

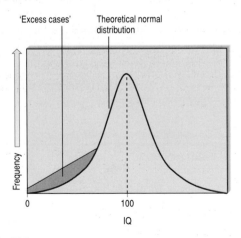

Figure 12.1
Frequency distribution in intelligence quotients (IQ). (Reproduced with permission from Puri BK, Laking PJ, Treasaden IH 1996 Textbook of psychiatry. Edinburgh: Churchill Livingstone.)

MILD MENTAL RETARDATION
Self-care and living skills

Most achieve full independence in self-care (eating, washing, dressing, bladder and bowel control). They may marry and hold down a job.

Language and communication skills

Most can use speech for normal circumstances and can hold conversations.

Education

Many have difficulties with reading and writing, but they can benefit from special education that aims to develop their skills.

MODERATE MENTAL RETARDATION
Self-care and living skills

Achievement of self-care and motor skills is retarded, but individuals are often able to attain considerable independence in daily living with some supervision. Some adults can carry out simple practical work.

Language and communication skills

The development of comprehension and use of language is slow and the eventual attainment limited. However, individuals are usually able to communicate adequately.

Education

Limited progress with school work is the norm, but special education that aims to develop the limited potential can be beneficial.

SEVERE MENTAL RETARDATION
Self-care and living skills

Achievement of self-care and motor skills is markedly retarded and many individuals require a great deal of help and supervision.

Language and communication skills

The development of comprehension and use of language is very limited and communication is often not by speech.

Education

There is very limited progress with school work.

....

PROFOUND MENTAL RETARDATION
Self-care and living skills

There is a severely limited ability to care for their own basic needs. Constant help and supervision is required.

Language and communication skills

The comprehension of language is severely limited. Most are able to communicate only in a very limited non-verbal way.

Education

This is extremely limited.

Table 12.3 Proportion of cases of mental retardation made up by each type

Degree of mental retardation	Proportion of all cases of mental retardation (%)
Mild	75
Moderate	20
Severe	5
Profound	< 1

....

PHYSICAL DISORDERS

Epilepsy, motor disorders (e.g. spasticity, ataxia and athetosis), speech defects and sensory disorders (e.g. visual and auditory defects) are more common in people with learning disabilities.

PSYCHIATRIC DISORDERS

The symptoms of psychiatric disorders are often altered in their presentation.

Schizophrenia

Poverty of thought is more common. Delusions and hallucinations tend to be less complex. The motor disturbances of schizophrenia may appear similar to those seen in non-psychotic mental retardation.

Mood disorder

Diurnal variation of mood may present as diurnal variation of behavioural disturbance. Other biological symptoms are usually a good guide to the presence of a mood disorder.

AETIOLOGY

Organic brain pathology is often present in those with an IQ of less than 50, but tends to be uncommon in the mildly mentally handicapped. The frequencies of the more common or well known conditions associated with mental retardation are shown in Figure 12.2

Down's syndrome

This is a common cause of mental retardation, with an incidence of between 1 in 600 and 1 in 700 live births; 95% of cases result from trisomy 21 following non-disjunction during meiosis, 4% are caused by translocation involving chromosome 21, and the remainder are mosaics. The majority of Down's syndrome babies are born to mothers aged over 35 (Figure 12.3).

Down's syndrome is characterized by bradycephaly, widely spaced eyes with epicanthic folds and oblique palpebral fissures, Brushfield spots, a small nose and mouth, a horizontally furrowed tongue, a high arched palate, malformed ears, broadening and shortening of the neck and hands, a single transverse palmar crease, curvature of the fifth finger, increased range of joint

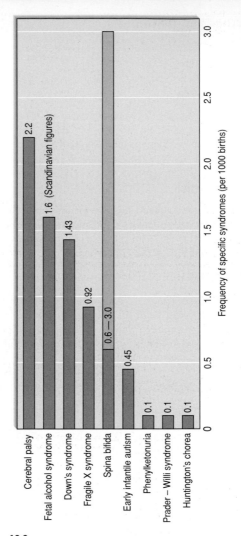

Figure 12.2
Frequencies (per 1000 births) of specific syndromes that may be associated with mental retardation. (Reproduced with permission from Puri BK, Laking PJ, Treasaden IH 1996 Textbook of psychiatry. Edinburgh: Churchill Livingstone.)

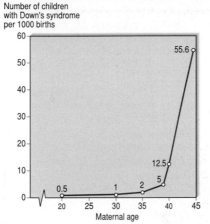

Figure 12.3
Incidence of Down's syndrome with increasing maternal age. (Reproduced with permission from Puri BK, Laking PJ, Treasaden IH 1996 Textbook of psychiatry. Edinburgh: Churchill Livingstone.)

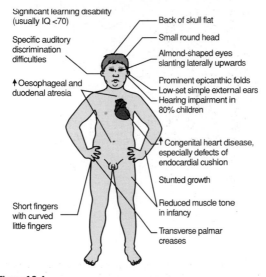

Figure 12.4
Clinical features of Down's syndrome. (Reproduced with permission from Puri BK, Laking PJ, Treasaden IH 1996 Textbook of psychiatry. Edinburgh: Churchill Livingstone.)

movements and hypotonia (Figure 12.4). It is associated with an increased incidence of cataracts, epilepsy, congenital cardiac disease, umbilical herniae, respiratory infections and acute leukaemia.

Fragile X syndrome

This is commoner in males, affecting 0.1% and associated with large floppy ears, prognathism and macro-orchidism (Figure 12.5). Female carriers have an increased likelihood of having poor muscular tone, joint hyperextensibility, prominent ears and elongated facies; one-third has reduced intellectual functioning.

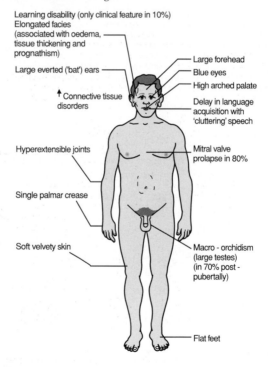

Figure 12.5
Clinical features of Fragile X syndrome. (Reproduced with permission from Puri BK, Laking PJ, Treasaden IH 1996 Textbook of psychiatry. Edinburgh: Churchill Livingstone.)

Childhood autism (Kanner's syndrome)

This is characterized by a general and profound failure to develop social relationships (autistic aloneness), speech and language retardation, ritualistic and compulsive behaviour, and an onset before the age of 30 months (Figure 12.6). It has a prevalence of 2 per 10 000 children in the community. When those with severe mental retardation are included the prevalence is increased. Autism can occur in association with all levels of IQ, but significant learning disability (mental retardation) occurs in about 75% of cases.

Other less common causes of mental retardation are included in Table 12.4.

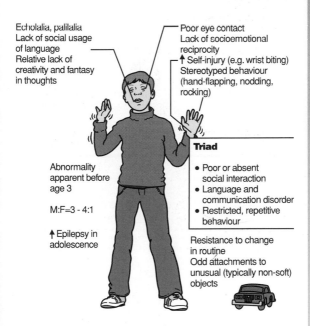

Echolalia, palilalia
Lack of social usage
of language
Relative lack of
creativity and fantasy
in thoughts

Poor eye contact
Lack of socioemotional
reciprocity
↑ Self-injury (e.g. wrist biting)
Stereotyped behaviour
(hand-flapping, nodding,
rocking)

Abnormality
apparent before
age 3

M:F=3 - 4:1

↑ Epilepsy in
adolescence

Triad

• Poor or absent
  social interaction
• Language and
  communication disorder
• Restricted, repetitive
  behaviour

Resistance to change
in routine
Odd attachments to
unusual (typically non-soft)
objects

Figure 12.6
Clinical features of childhood autism (Kanner's syndrome). (Reproduced with permission from Puri BK, Laking PJ, Treasaden IH 1996 Textbook of psychiatry. Edinburgh: Churchill Livingstone.)

Table 12.4 Causes of learning disabilities

Genetic	
Autosomal dominant	Phakomatoses (tuberous sclerosis, neurofibromatosis, von Hippel–Lindau syndrome, Sturge–Weber syndrome), Huntington's disease, acrocallosal syndrome
Autosomal recessive	Phenylketonuria, homocystinuria, galactosaemia, Tay–Sachs disease, Hurler's syndrome
X-linked	Fragile X syndrome, Lesch–Nyhan syndrome, Rett's syndrome
Chromosome abnormalities	Down's syndrome, Edward's syndrome, Patau's syndrome, *cri du chat* syndrome, triple-X syndrome
Maternal infection	Rubella during the first 16 weeks of pregnancy, toxoplasmosis, cytomegalovirus, congenital syphilis, listeriosis
Childhood infection	Encephalitis, meningitis
Cranial malformation	Hydrocephalus, microcephaly
Nutritional and toxic causes	Placental dysfunction, malnutrition, hypoglycaemia, fetal alcohol syndrome, lead intoxication
Anoxia	
Traumatic	Accidental injury, child abuse, perinatal trauma

Psychiatry of the elderly

The proportion of the population that is elderly is predicted to continue to increase rapidly in many countries. For example, in the USA the number of people aged 85 and over was 3.3 million in 1990, and this is expected to increase to 12.8 million by 2040. A quarter of those aged 65 and over suffer from psychiatric disorders, most commonly dementia and depression.

SERVICES FOR THE ELDERLY

The development of psychiatric services for the elderly has been particularly strong in the British National Health Service. Everyone in a given catchment area over a given age is dealt with by a multidisciplinary team, which includes psychiatrists and community psychiatric nurses. This offers domiciliary assessments, community nursing, day hospital care, respite inpatient admissions, and liaison with physicians who look after the elderly.

PSYCHIATRIC DISORDERS
Delirium

Delirium is relatively common in the elderly, who are prone to physical disorders.

Dementia

Dementia is increasingly prevalent with increasing age. The most common dementia in the elderly is Alzheimer's disease, followed by multi-infarct dementia. Depressive pseudodementia should be borne in mind as an important differential diagnosis in this age group.

The management of dementia should include:

- Regular respite inpatient admissions to support carers
- Community psychiatric nurse support and liaison with GPs and psychiatrists
- Occupational therapy to help in assessing and encouraging the patient's potential abilities
- Reality orientation and reminiscence therapy
- Sheltered accommodation or a long-stay inpatient ward may be required as the dementia progresses
- Regular appointments with an optician for the early detection of cataracts and glaucoma
- Regular appointments with a dentist to check dental health and replace unsatisfactory dentures, if necessary
- Chiropody for those unable to look after their own feet
- Physiotherapy to help with mobility, and muscle and joint-related pain relief
- Continence advisers can assess, advise and sometimes treat urinary and faecal incontinence
- Attendance, mobility and invalid care allowances are available in many countries
- Attendance at a day hospital and/or local authority day centre.

Non-statutory voluntary agencies are a valuable source of support. In Britain these include Age Concern, the Alzheimer's Disease Society, Help the Aged, and Citizens' Advice Bureaux. Local schemes include sitting services, visiting and befriending groups, sheltered housing schemes, and talking newspaper and book services.

In due course useful pharmacological treatments may become available as a result of the research effort currently being undertaken.

Depression

Depressed elderly patients may present atypically with:

- Agitated depression
- Symptoms masked by concurrent physical illness
- Minimization or denial of low mood
- Hypochondriasis
- Complaints of loneliness

- Complaints disproportionate to organic pathology and pain of unknown origin
- Onset of neurotic symptoms
- Depressive pseudodementia
- Behavioural disturbance (e.g. food refusal, aggressive behaviour, shoplifting, alcohol abuse).

Pharmacotherapy with antidepressants is usually the first-line treatment. In resistant cases a course of electroconvulsive therapy (ECT) may give a good response. Socially isolated elderly depressed patients have a high suicide risk and should be treated energetically.

Differentiating between pseudodementia (depression) and dementia (Alzheimer's disease)

Pseudodementia, a term used to describe a presentation which is that of an organic dementia but where there is also a functional disorder, can result from any functional disorder. In practice depression is considered to be the disorder present. Table 13.1 summarizes important differences between pseudodementia and dementia.

Paraphrenia

In ICD-10 'paraphrenia (late)' is included within 'delusional disorder'. Delusional disorders in the elderly are particularly likely to occur in those who live alone and have sensory deprivation, e.g. from poor eyesight or hearing. An elderly patient presenting with a delusional disorder should therefore have their eyesight and hearing checked. The mainstay of treatment is antipsychotic medication, which should be given in low doses. Social services intervention and day hospital attendance can help with social isolation.

··

MEDICATION
Side-effects of drugs

Side-effects should be carefully considered before medications are prescribed to the elderly. For example, antipsychotics and tricyclic antidepressants can cause

Table 13.1 Differentiation of pseudodementia and dementia

	Pseudodementia (depression)	Dementia (Alzheimer's disease)
History		
Onset	Can usually be dated accurately	Usually unclear
Progress of symptoms	Rapid	Slow
Family psychiatric history of depression	More common	Less common
Past psychiatric history of depression	More common	Less common
Complaints of memory loss by patient	Common	Rare
Disabilities	Often emphasized by the patient	Often concealed by the patient
Mental state examination		
Appearance and behaviour	Patients tend to convey their distress	Patients tend not to convey their distress
Mood	Depressed	May be labile
Replies to questions	Often reply 'I don't know'	Tend to be incorrect
Specific memory gaps	More common	Less common
Task performance	Little effort may be made	The patient may try hard
Special investigations		
MRI or CT	Little evidence of cerebral atrophy - usually exists	Cerebral atrophy and ventricular enlargement
EEG	Usually normal	Pronounced slow wave activity common
SPECT	Normal rCBF patterns usual	Parietotemporal and frontal deficits common

postural hypotension, which may cause the patient to fall and suffer a fracture. The side effect of dry mouth may make it difficult for elderly patients to wear dentures. Urinary retention may lead to anuria. Cardiovascular side effects may cause myocardial or cerebral infarction. Central antimuscarinic side effects, such as impaired concentration and memory, and delirium, are dangerous in the elderly.

Polypharmacy

Polypharmacy often occurs in the elderly, leading to an increased risk of side effects and non-compliance. Therefore, a careful review of the medication should be carried out.

Sedatives and anxiolytics

In many countries sedatives and anxiolytics, including those of the benzodiazepine group, are overprescribed to the elderly. In addition to problems of dependency, increased sensitivity in this age group leads to an increased risk of postural instability, hangover sedation, and impairment of cognitive and psychomotor performance.

Drugs for dementia

Anticholinesterase inhibitors may be used for cognitive enhancement in mild to moderate Alzheimer's disease. Cognitive assessment is repeated at around 3 months, and if the patient is not responding the anticholinesterase inhibitor should be discontinued; up to 50% of patients show a slowed rate of cognitive decline. Many specialists repeat the cognitive assessment 4–6 weeks after discontinuation to confirm lack of deterioration.

Donepezil This is a reversible acetylcholinesterase inhibitor that is hepatically metabolized. It may cause unwanted cholinergic side effects.

Rivastigmine This is a reversible non-competitive acetylcholinesterase inhibitor. It may cause unwanted cholinergic side effects.

Suicide and parasuicide

An understanding of the differences between those who commit suicide and those who survive following self-harm (parasuicide or deliberate self-harm) is essential in order to be able to assess suicide risk.

SUICIDE

Epidemiology

Sex ratio
Commoner in males.

Age
Commoner in those aged over 45 years.

Marriage
Highest rates in those who are divorced, single or widowed. Those who are married have the lowest rate.

Social class
Highest rates in social classes I and V.

Employment
Associated with lack of employment, including both unemployment and retirement.

Season
Highest rates in spring and early summer.

Aetiology

Psychiatric disorder

This is present in 90% of those who commit suicide, particularly:

- Depressive episodes: many actually use their antidepressants (tricyclics and MAOIs) to kill themselves with – the newer antidepressants (SSRI, RIMA, NARI, SNRI and NaSSA groups) are much safer in overdosage
- Alcohol dependence
- Illicit drug abuse
- Personality disorder
- Chronic neuroses
- Schizophrenia, particularly in young men with low mood.

Physical illness

Suicide is associated with:

- Chronic painful illnesses
- Epilepsy.

Parasuicide

Following an act of parasuicide the risk of committing suicide in the following year is approximately 100 times that in the general population.

Assessment

It is important to ask about any suicidal thoughts (there is no evidence that such questions might introduce the idea of suicide and precipitate such action). If there is any evidence of such thoughts the reasons for them and the methods being considered should be explored.

Any statement to the effect that there is no future or that suicide is being considered should be taken very seriously. The majority of those who commit suicide have told someone beforehand of their thoughts; two-thirds have seen their GP in the previous month. A quarter are psychiatric outpatients at the time of death; half of them will have seen a psychiatrist in the previous week.

Evidence of the psychiatric and physical illnesses mentioned above should be looked for, as should evidence of loneliness and reduced or no social contacts. Relatives and friends should also be interviewed and information obtained about any losses, such as the break-up of a relationship, death of a relative or close friend, loss of job, financial loss, or loss of status in society (e.g. after being arrested for shoplifting).

Management

If there is a serious risk of suicide the patient should be admitted to hospital, compulsorily if need be. A good rapport should be established between patient and staff so that the patient feels free to articulate his or her feelings and suicidal thoughts. Any potentially lethal implements (e.g. sharp objects and belts) should be removed. The patient may need to be observed continuously and be nursed in pyjamas (without a cord) or a nightdress throughout the day.

Any psychiatric disorder should be treated appropriately. For a severe depressive episode ECT may be required, as this will act faster than antidepressant treatment.

PARASUICIDE (DELIBERATE SELF-HARM)

Parasuicide is any self-initiated act deliberately undertaken by a patient who mimics the act of suicide, but which does not result in a fatal outcome. It is an act in which the patient injures himself or herself, or takes a substance in a quantity which exceeds the therapeutic dose (if any) or his or her habitual level of consumption, and which he or she believes to be pharmacologically active.

Methods used

In the UK 90% of cases involve deliberate self-poisoning with drugs. In many cases these are prescribed drugs, such as antidepressants. Paracetamol, which is freely obtainable, is particularly dangerous as an overdose of as little as 10 g can lead to severe hepatocellular necrosis; patients who change their mind after taking the overdose, or who had not really wished to die, may go on to develop encephalopathy, haemorrhage and cerebral oedema within a few days, and then die.

Epidemiology

Sex ratio

Commoner in females.

Age

Commoner in those aged below 45 years, particularly those between 15 and 25.

Marriage

Highest rates in those who are divorced, single or teenage wives.

Social class

Highest rates in the lower social classes.

Employment

Associated with unemployment.

Geographical

Commoner in urban areas in which there is:

- High unemployment
- Overcrowding
- High social mobility
- High rates of juvenile delinquency
- High rates of sexually transmitted diseases.

Aetiology

Life events

Compared with the general population, life events are more common in the 6 months before an act of parasuicide, e.g.:

- The break-up of a relationship
- Being in trouble with the law
- Physical illness
- Illness of a loved one.

Predisposing factors

These include:

- Marital difficulties, e.g. infidelity
- Unemployment
- Physical illness, particularly epilepsy
- Mental retardation

PUERPERAL PSYCHOSIS
Clinical features

Three types of psychotic disorder can occur following childbirth: affective, schizophrenic and acute organic.

Epidemiology
Rate
About 1 in 500 live births.

Onset
Usually between day 3 and day 14 postpartum.

Prevalence of subtypes
Affective (70–80%) and schizophrenic (20–25%). Organic psychoses are now very rare in the West.

Previous pregnancies
Commoner in primigravidae.

Aetiology

The predisposing causes include those for non-puerperal psychotic disorders, particularly genetic factors. It may be that endocrine changes following childbirth act as a precipitating factor.

Management
Hospitalization
This is usually required, preferably in a mother and baby unit so that the baby can be cared for by the nursing staff when the mother is too ill, and by the mother when she is better. The close proximity of the baby to the mother helps encourage bonding and diminishes feelings of guilt in the mother.

Treatment
This is as described in earlier chapters. If a drug given to the mother is excreted in significant amounts in breast milk, then breastfeeding may have to be stopped. Electroconvulsive therapy (ECT) may need to be given in cases of severe depression because of its rapid action, thereby allowing the mother to resume caring for her baby sooner.

Prognosis

Most recover fully; the affective type has a better prognosis than the schizophrenic type. The recurrence rate of a puerperal psychosis is 14–20%. The risk of a non-puerperal psychotic disorder may be as high as 50%.

....

POSTNATAL DEPRESSION
Clinical features

Non-psychotic depression is the most important puerperal neurosis and may manifest as excessive anxiety about the baby's health, self-blame, sleep disturbance, depressive symptoms, suicidal thoughts, fear of harming the baby, or rejection of the baby.

Epidemiology
Rate
Ten to 15% of mothers.

Onset
Usually 2–6 weeks postpartum.

Previous pregnancies
No association.

Aetiology

A past psychiatric history and recent life stressful events may predispose; emotional instability during the first postpartum week is associated with a greater risk of developing postnatal depression.

Management

This includes antidepressant medication, reassurance and counselling.

Prognosis

Ninety per cent of cases last less than 1 month; about 4% are still depressed 1 year postpartum.

Treatments

In clinical practice it is helpful to consider types of treatment under the headings physical, psychological and social.

PHYSICAL TREATMENTS
Pharmacotherapy (drug treatment)

As mentioned in the preface, it is highly recommended that the reader always refer to the most up-to-date formulary available when prescribing drugs. (In Britain, this is the most recent edition of the *British National Formulary*.)

Antipsychotic drugs (neuroleptics)
Main uses
The treatment of schizophrenia, the acute symptoms of mania, and psychotic symptoms arising from organic disorders and psychoactive substance use.

Examples
Typical (standard) antipsychotics include chlorpromazine, haloperidol, trifluoperazine, droperidol, fluphenazine, zuclopenthixol and flupenthixol. Atypical antipsychotics include clozapine, risperidone, amisulpiride, olanzapine, quetiapine and zotepine.

Mode of action
Typical antipsychotics cause central postsynaptic blockade of dopamine D_2 receptors. Atypical antipsychotics have a much greater action than do typical antipsychotics on other receptors, such as other dopamine receptors and serotonin (5-HT) receptors.

Administration
Oral, intramuscular and rectal suppositories are available for chlorpromazine. Slow-release depot preparations

administered by deep intramuscular injection, usually at intervals of 2–8 weeks, are available (e.g. flupenthixol decanoate, fluphenazine decanoate, haloperidol decanoate and zuclopenthixol decanoate).

Main side-effects

The antidopaminergic action on the tuberoinfundibular system leads to hyperprolactinaemia, which in turn causes galactorrhoea, gynaecomastia, menstrual disturbances, reduced sperm count and reduced libido.

The antidopaminergic action on the nigrostriatal system leads to extrapyramidal side-effects (parkinsonism, dystonias, akathisia and tardive dyskinesia). Atypical antipsychotics have a low propensity to cause extrapyramidal side-effects. (An important side effect of clozapine is neutropenia, and so regular haematological monitoring is required.)

Peripheral antimuscarinic (anticholinergic) actions lead to dry mouth, blurred vision, urinary retention and constipation.

Central antimuscarinic actions lead to convulsions and pyrexia.

Antiadrenergic actions lead to postural hypotension and failure of ejaculation.

Antihistaminic actions lead to drowsiness.

The most serious side effect is the neuroleptic malignant syndrome, a rare but potentially fatal toxic delirious state characterized by hyperthermia, a fluctuating level of consciousness, muscular rigidity and autonomic dysfunction (tachycardia, labile blood pressure, pallor, sweating and urinary incontinence); abnormal investigation results include increased creatinine phosphokinase, increased WBC and abnormal liver function tests. Neuroleptic malignant syndrome requires urgent medical treatment.

Long-term high-dose treatment leads to eye and skin changes (e.g. opacities of the lens and cornea) and a purplish pigmentation of the skin, conjunctiva, cornea and retina.

Antimuscarinic (anticholinergic) drugs
Main uses

The treatment of parkinsonian symptoms resulting from antipsychotic pharmacotherapy. They should not be prescribed routinely, but only if parkinsonism occurs.

Examples

Procyclidine, benzhexol, benztropine and orphenadrine.

Mode of action

Antimuscarinic action.

Administration

Procyclidine and benztropine can be administered orally, intramuscularly and intravenously. Parenteral administration is used in acute dystonic reactions (tongue protrusion, grimacing, opisthotonus, spasmodic torticollis or oculogyric crisis).

Main side effects

Antimuscarinic (see above). They can also worsen tardive dyskinesia and affect memory.

Lithium salts

Main uses

The prophylaxis of bipolar mood disorder and recurrent depression. The treatment of resistant depression, (hypo)mania, aggression and self-mutilation. (Antipsychotics act more rapidly than lithium in the treatment of (hypo)mania.)

Examples

Lithium carbonate and lithium citrate.

Administration

Oral.

Monitoring

Renal function must be checked before starting lithium, as the drug is excreted by the kidneys.

Once on treatment, regular monitoring of plasma levels is required (these should be between 0.4 and 1.0 mmol/l, 8–12 hours post dose, for prophylactic purposes) because of its low therapeutic/toxic ratio. Urea, electrolytes and the creatinine level must also be regularly monitored to check renal function. Thyroid function tests should be checked regularly because thyroid function disturbances can result from long-term lithium therapy.

Main side-effects

Gastrointestinal side-effects, fine tremor, dry mouth, poly-uria, polydipsia, weight gain and oedema (see Figure 16.1).

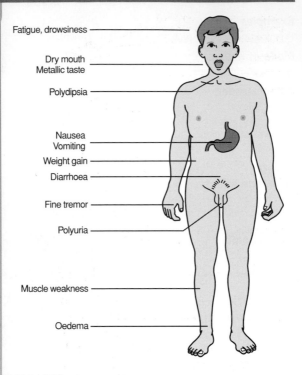

Figure 16.1
Side-effects of lithium (Reproduced with permission from Puri BK, Laking PJ, Treasaden IH 1996 Textbook of psychiatry. Edinburgh: Churchill Livingstone.)

Oedema should not be treated with diuretics because thiazide and loop diuretics reduce lithium excretion and so can cause lithium intoxication.

Signs of lithium intoxication are shown in Figure 16.2.

At plasma levels above 2 mmol/l the following effects occur: hyperreflexia and hyperextension of limbs, toxic psychoses, convulsions, syncope, oliguria, circulatory failure, coma and death.

Long-term treatment can lead to thyroid function disturbances (goitre, hypothyroidism, hyperthyroidism), memory impairment, nephrotoxicity and cardiovascular changes (T-wave flattening and arrhythmias).

It is useful to give the patient a lithium card describing the side-effects, how to take the lithium, the need for regular

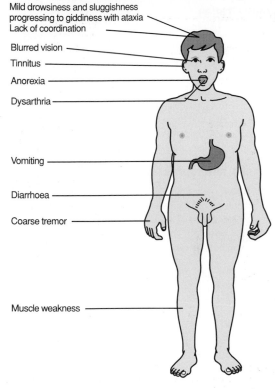

Mild drowsiness and sluggishness
progressing to giddiness with ataxia
Lack of coordination

Blurred vision

Tinnitus

Anorexia

Dysarthria

Vomiting

Diarrhoea

Coarse tremor

Muscle weakness

Figure 16.2
Signs of lithium intoxication (Reproduced with permission from Puri BK,
Laking PJ, Treasaden IH 1996 Textbook of psychiatry. Edinburgh: Churchill
Livingstone.)

blood monitoring, and the need to keep up an adequate
fluid intake and avoid dietary changes that may cause
changes in the sodium intake.

Carbamazepine

Main uses

Instead of, or in combination with, lithium in cases of
bipolar affective (mood) disorder resistant to lithium,
resistant mania and resistant depression. Also used in
epilepsy and trigeminal neuralgia.

Administration
Oral.

Monitoring
The full blood count and liver function tests should be checked before starting the drug. Once started, regular monitoring of the plasma carbamazepine level allows the optimum dosage to be determined. The full blood count should be checked regularly because carbamazepine may depress the WBC.

Tricyclic antidepressants

Main uses
The treatment of depressive illness, obsessive–compulsive disorder, generalized anxiety disorder, panic disorder and phobic disorders. In children they are used in low doses to treat nocturnal enuresis.

Examples
Imipramine (less sedating), amitripyline (more sedating), clomipramine and lofepramine (less toxic).

Mode of action
The antidepressant action results from inhibiting the reuptake of the monoamines noradrenaline and serotonin (5-HT), hence the acronym MARIs (MonoAmine Reuptake Inhibitors).

Their use in treating enuresis is a result of their antimuscarinic action leading to urinary retention.

Administration
Usually orally. Preparations for intramuscular and intravenous administration are also available for some tricyclic antidepressants.

Main side-effects
Peripheral and central antimuscarinic side-effects (e.g. dry mouth, blurred vision, constipation, urinary retention, sedation and nausea).

Cardiovascular side-effects include ECG changes (T-wave flattening, prolongation of QT interval and ST depression), postural hypotension and arrhythmias.

Other side-effects are shown in Figure 16.3.

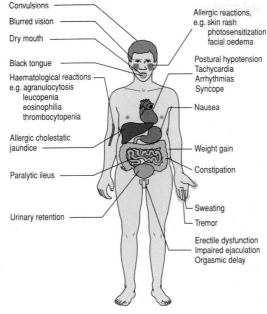

Figure 16.3
Side effects of tricyclic antidepressants (Reproduced with permission from Puri BK, Laking PJ, Treasaden IH 1996 Textbook of psychiatry. Edinburgh: Churchill Livingstone.)

In overdose tricyclic antidepressants are toxic, causing cardiac conduction defects, arrhythmias, convulsions, respiratory failure, coma and death.

Selective serotonin reuptake inhibitors (SSRIs)

Main uses
The treatment of depressive illness, obsessive–compulsive disorder, bulimia nervosa, panic disorder and phobic disorders.

Examples
Fluvoxamine, fluoxetine, paroxetine, sertraline and citalopram.

Mode of action
Selective central inhibition of the reuptake of serotonin (5-HT).

Administration

Oral.

Main side-effects

Gastrointestinal (nausea, vomiting and diarrhoea) owing to action on gut 5-HT receptors. Occasionally they cause sexual dysfunction, particularly delayed ejaculation.

They are safe in overdose.

Selective noradrenaline and serotonin reuptake inhibitor (SNRI)

Main uses

The treatment of depressive illness.

Example

Venlafaxine.

Mode of action

Selective central inhibition of the reuptake of noradrenaline and serotonin (5-HT).

Administration

Oral.

Main side-effects

Similar profile to that of SSRIs. At higher doses hypertension may occur.

Selective noradrenaline reuptake inhibitor (NARI)

Main uses

The treatment of depressive illness.

Example

Reboxetine.

Mode of action

Selective central inhibition of the reuptake of noradrenaline.

Administration

Oral.

Main side effects

Dry mouth, constipation, increased sweating, insomnia, postural hypotension and urinary retention (mainly in men).

Noradrenergic and specific serotonergic antidepressant (NaSSA)

Main uses
The treatment of depressive illness.

Example
Mirtazapine.

Mode of action
Increases central noradrenaline release by antagonizing inhibitory presynaptic α_2-adrenoceptors. It also increases serotonin release by both enhancing a facilitatory noradrenergic input to serotonergic cell bodies and antagonizing inhibitory presynaptic α_2-adrenoceptors on serotonergic neuronal terminals.

Administration
Oral.

Main side-effects
Sedation (usually in the first few weeks of treatment), increased appetite and weight gain. Relatively safe in overdose.

Monoamine oxidase inhibitors (MAOIs)

Main uses
The treatment of depression refractory to other antidepressants; depression with severe anxiety, atypical, hypochondriacal or hysterical features; phobic disorders with atypical, hypochondriacal or hysterical features; agoraphobia; and obsessive–compulsive disorder.

Examples
Phenelzine, isocarboxazid and tranylcypromine.

Mode of action
The inhibition of the metabolic degradation of monoamines by monoamine oxidase.

Administration
Oral.

Main side-effects
MAOIs interact dangerously with tyramine-containing foods by inhibiting the peripheral metabolism of pressor

amines. Dietary tyramine can lead to a hypertensive crisis ('cheese reaction') in patients being treated with MAOIs. Foods which should therefore be avoided include:

- Cheese (*except* cottage cheese and cream cheese)
- Meat extracts and yeast extracts (e.g. Bovril, Marmite, Oxo)
- Alcohol (particularly Chianti, fortified wines and beer)
- Herring (pickled or smoked)
- Non-fresh fish, meat or poultry (e.g. seasoned game)
- Offal
- Avocado
- Banana skins
- Broad bean pods
- Caviar.

Indirectly acting sympathomimetic amines (e.g. those found in cough mixtures and nasal decongestants) must also be avoided.

Tricyclic antidepressants can interact dangerously with MAOIs: for example, deaths have resulted from the combination of tranylcypromine with clomipramine.

After stopping treatment with a MAOI 2 weeks should elapse before starting a tricyclic antidepressant or SSRI or related antidepressant (NARI, SNRI, NaSSA), and before it is safe to take any of the above forbidden foodstuffs and medicines.

For a patient first treated with an SSRI or related antidepressant (NARI, SNRI, NaSSA), 2–5 weeks (depending on the SSRI) must elapse before a MAOI can be started.

Other side-effects include antimuscarinic actions, hepatotoxicity, appetite stimulation and weight gain. Tranylcypromine may cause dependency.

MAOI treatment cards listing precautions to be taken should be given to patients.

Reversible inhibitor of monoamine oxidase-A (RIMA)

Main uses

As for MAOIs; also the treatment of social phobia.

Example

Moclobemide.

Mode of action
The selective and reversible inhibition of the metabolic degradation of monoamines by monoamine oxidase type A (MAO-A).

Administration
Oral.

Main side-effects
Because they are reversible RIMAs can be displaced by other substances, such as tyramine, and are therefore much less likely to cause a food or drug interaction than are MAOIs. A few patients may be especially sensitive to tyramine, and therefore all patients are advised not to consume large quantities of tyramine-rich foodstuffs or to use sympathomimetics.

Benzodiazepines
Main uses
The short-term relief (2–4 weeks) of severe or disabling anxiety. The short-term treatment of insomnia, only when it is severe or disabling. Benzodiazepines are also used as anticonvulsants, as muscle relaxants, as premedication in anaesthesia, in the immediate treatment of aggressive behaviour, and in the treatment of alcohol dependence.

Examples
- Long-acting: chlordiazepoxide, diazepam and nitrazepam.
- Short-acting: lorazepam, lormetazepam and temazepam.

Mode of action
They bind to central benzodiazepine receptors linked to GABA (γ-aminobutyric acid) receptors in a complex involving GABA and benzodiazepine receptors and a chloride channel.

Administration
Oral, intravenous, rectal and intramuscular preparations are available for many benzodiazepines.

Main side-effects
Psychomotor impairment.

Long-acting benzodiazepines are likely to cause hangover-like effects if used as hypnotics. Short-acting ones are more likely to cause withdrawal effects.

If taken regularly for at least 4 weeks dependence may develop. When regular intake is stopped suddenly the benzodiazepine withdrawal syndrome occurs, which may include insomnia, anxiety symptoms, low mood, depersonalization, derealization, distorted perception of space, tinnitus, formication, influenza-like symptoms, loss of appetite and weight, seizures, confusional states and psychotic episodes.

In overdose the benzodiazepines taken alone are safe, causing drowsiness or sleep.

Azaspirodecanedione

Main uses
The short-term treatment of anxiety disorders and the relief of anxiety symptoms.

Example
Buspirone.

Mode of action
Acts as a central 5-HT$_{1A}$ partial agonist.

Administration
Oral.

Main side-effects
Dizziness, headache, excitement and nausea. It does not cause dependence.

Drugs used in alcohol dependence

Benzodiazepines and chlormethiazole, given in a reducing regimen, are used in the management of alcohol withdrawal symptoms.

Disulfiram is used in prophylactic adjunctive pharmaco-therapy to prevent alcohol intake. When taken regularly it causes acetaldehyde to accumulate in the body if alcohol is ingested, leading to unpleasant systemic reactions (see Chapter 4).

The use of acamprosate is described in Chapter 4.

Drugs used in opioid dependence

Methadone is an opioid agonist that can be used to reduce withdrawal symptoms in opioid dependence by substituting for the opioid. Naltrexone is an opioid antagonist that can be used as an adjunct to prevent relapse following detoxification.

Cyproterone acetate

Cyproterone acetate is an antiandrogen that can be used to control libido in severe hypersexuality and/or sexual deviation in men. Its mode of action is shown in Figure 16.4.

Electroconvulsive therapy (ECT)
Main uses

The treatment, in cases in which drug treatment is too slow or the patient resistant to drugs, of severe depressive illness (e.g. when there is a high immediate risk of suicide or

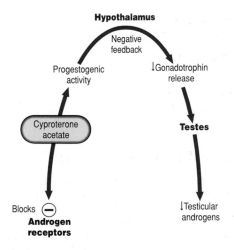

Figure 16.4
The antiandrogen actions of cyproterone acetate. (Reproduced with permission from Puri BK, Laking PJ, Treasaden IH 1996 Textbook of psychiatry. Edinburgh: Churchill Livingstone.)

insufficient fluid intake to maintain renal function), puerperal depressive illness, mania, catatonic schizophrenia and schizoaffective disorder.

Administration

Bilaterally, or unilaterally to the non-dominant cerebral hemisphere.

Main side-effects

Early side-effects include headache, temporary confusion and some loss of short-term memory (greater following bilateral ECT).

Depressed patients with bipolar affective (mood) disorder may become manic.

In the long-term bilateral ECT is more likely than unilateral ECT to lead to complaints of impaired memory (not generally borne out by objective testing).

Contraindications

Raised intracranial pressure and other physical disorders (e.g. cerebral aneurysm, recent myocardial infarction and cardiac arrhythmia) that may be worsened by the blood pressure rise caused by ECT. Other contraindications include physical disorders that make anaesthesia risky (e.g. cardiac disease and chest infection).

Psychosurgery

Main uses

It is used very rarely, as a last resort in treating chronic severe intractable depression and obsessive–compulsive disorder, when all other treatments have failed.

Administration

Stereotaxic lesions can be made using electrocautery, radioactive yttrium implantation, and thermocoagulation.

....

PSYCHOLOGICAL TREATMENTS
Behaviour therapy

Behaviour therapy is a brief goal-directed psychological treatment based on behavioural learning theory, dealing with the current features of the disorder and involving a continued objective assessment of progress.

Systematic desensitization

Graded exposure, either in reality or in imagination, takes place in conjunction with relaxation training. It can be used to treat phobic disorders.

Flooding

The patient is subjected to the stimulus all at once, and this is repeated until there is no longer any anxiety. It can be used to treat phobic disorders.

Response prevention

In the treatment of obsessive–compulsive disorder, carrying out rituals is repeatedly prevented and the corresponding distress gradually diminishes.

Modelling

The patient physically follows the example of the therapist. It can be used to treat phobic disorders and compulsive rituals (e.g. concerning contamination).

Thought stopping

Unwanted thoughts are interrupted by thinking or saying 'STOP' whenever the unwanted thought occurs; at first a rubber band worn around the wrist can also be snapped against the wrist when the unwanted thought occurs. It can be used to treat obsessional thoughts.

Assertiveness training

Roles are acted out in imaginary situations replicating circumstances found difficult in real life, using role-playing, role-reversal, modelling and coaching. It can be used to treat social phobia and shyness.

Social skills training

Role-playing, role-reversal, modelling, coaching and video feedback can be used to treat those with poor social skills.

Token economy

A system based on operant conditioning in which tokens given to reward desired behaviours become a secondary reinforcer (the tokens can be exchanged for goods or privileges). It can be used to alter the behaviour of long-stay patients and hostel residents with chronic schizophrenia or learning disability.

Bell-and-pad method

This can be used to treat nocturnal enuresis. A bell rings when bedwetting starts and the child has to get up and use the lavatory; in time, the bedwetting may stop.

Aversion therapy

Negative reinforcement is used to prevent unsuitable thoughts or behaviour. It is now rarely used.

Cognitive therapy

Cognitive therapy is based on a model in which the processing of information is held to be of central importance and it is attempted to change this when treating psychiatric disorders. Disorders that have been found to respond include depression, phobic disorders, anxiety disorders and bulimia nervosa.

Maladaptive thoughts are elicited and challenged during therapy. Examples seen in depression include:

Arbitrary inference

The worst negative inferences are made arbitrarily from situations.

Catastrophizing

Errors are turned, cognitively, into catastrophes.

Dichotomous thinking

The attitudes of others are seen in a dichotomous way.

Maximization

The significance of negative events is maximized.

Minimization

The significance of positive events is minimized.

Overgeneralization

Overgeneralized inferences are made from one negative occurrence.

Personalization

Negative events are personalized to oneself, leading to guilt.

Selective abstraction

The negative aspects of any situation are selectively focused on.

Individual psychotherapy

Main aims
Symptom relief and personality change.

Main uses
The treatment of symptoms of neurotic disorders, such as anxiety disorders, hysterical conversion disorders and obsessive–compulsive disorder, and psychosomatic disorders.

Essential elements
These are free association, dream analysis, analysing transference and countertransference, working with the patient's resistance and defence mechanisms, and using clarification, linking, reflection, interpretation and confrontation.

Administration
Each session often lasts 50 minutes. Individual therapy may entail five sessions per week over many years.

Brief focal psychotherapy

This differs from individual long-term psychodynamic psychotherapy in that it is much briefer, a focus is selected to be worked on, and the ending of therapy may have to be worked with much sooner.

Group psychotherapy

This has similar aims to individual psychotherapy but is carried out in a group setting with more than one patient and one therapist.

Family therapy

A type of group psychotherapy used to treat family psychopathology in which the group consists of members of one family with one therapist or two co-therapists.

Marital therapy

This is offered to couples who seek and need help with relationship difficulties; behavioural models and contracts may be used.

Sex therapy

This is used in the treatment of a couple presenting with sexual dysfunction, and aims to enable individuals to feel at ease with their sexuality and to improve the quality of the couple's sexual relationship. Behavioural and psychotherapeutic techniques are used.

Art and music therapies

These allow the patient to express himself or herself in art and music, which take the place of verbal articulation in individual and group psychotherapies.

....

SOCIAL AND COMMUNITY ASPECTS
Occupational therapy

The patient or hostel resident is taught skills required for daily living (e.g. shopping, cooking, and organizing one's life better) which may have been lost (e.g. in chronic schizophrenia) or never developed (e.g. in learning disability).

Rehabilitation

Rehabilitation programmes are used in treating chronically ill patients (e.g. chronic schizophrenia) who find it difficult to live outside hospital. A detailed assessment of disabilities and potential abilities is followed by setting goals and designing a plan to reach them. The programme is modified as required according to the response.

Sheltered workshops

Specially set up subsidized places of employment where the chronically ill (e.g. chronic schizophrenia) can obtain work experience and an increased sense of self-worth, if they cannot obtain meaningful employment in the open market.

Sheltered accommodation

Specially set up subsidized places of residence where the chronically ill (e.g. chronic schizophrenia) can live outside hospital, if they cannot cope with living on their own in the community. Hostels may be run by psychiatrically qualified staff, allowing the mental state, physical health and medication of the resident to be monitored.

Early intervention services

Patients in the community can be treated by early intervention services, thereby possibly pre-empting the need for inpatient admission.

Social work

Social workers have multiple and increasingly complex roles in the social and community aspects of psychiatric treatment, including informal support, local service provision, the assessment of patients in the community with respect to legislation (for example, liaising with general practitioners and psychiatrists in the community in assessing whether individuals should be compulsorily admitted to hospital under mental health legislation), multiprofessional work in the community, and case management.

Environmental (community) interventions in families

Environmental interventions have been used particularly with the families of patients with schizophrenia. They may include: educating the family about the patient's disorder; working through problem-solving activities with families; improving communication; lowering expressed emotion (particularly in families of patients with schizophrenia); when appropriate, lowering expectations; reducing contact (for example, by placing patients with schizophrenia in sheltered daytime activities and encouraging patients and their relatives to pursue different leisure activities); and expanding the social networks of both patients and their relatives.

Transcultural psychiatry

Psychiatric disorders can have different presentations in different cultures. Furthermore, there are certain disorders, known as culture-bound syndromes, that occur only in certain cultural groups.

PRESENTATION OF PSYCHIATRIC DISORDERS

The presentation of psychiatric disorders in non-western populations, particularly in immigrants to western countries, can differ from that of the indigenous populations of western countries. It may be helpful to speak to an informant from the patient's community during assessment.

Depression

Depressed non-western immigrants to the west may not complain of depression. Afro-Caribbean men may complain instead of erectile dysfunction or reduced libido, whereas men and women from the Indian subcontinent may complain of somatic symptoms such as abdominal pains. Any physical disorder that may cause depressed mood, e.g. tuberculosis, should also be investigated.

Schizophrenia

Catatonic symptoms are commoner in some non-western countries. Those of Afro-Caribbean origin may believe in voodoo, so that the expression of such a belief may not be delusional.

CULTURE-BOUND SYNDROMES

These are specific disorders occurring in certain non-western countries (see Figure 17.1).

Amok

Amok is seen in southeast Asia. Following a depressive episode there is an outburst of aggressive behaviour in which the patient runs amok.

Koro

Koro is seen in southeast Asia, particularly in Malayans of Chinese extraction, and in parts of China. Affected men have an overwhelming fear that their penis is retracting into the abdomen and that death will then occur.

Latah

Latah is seen in the Far East and North Africa. It is a dissociative disorder in which patients exhibit echolalia, echopraxia and automatic obedience.

Piblokto

Piblokto is seen in Eskimo women. It is a dissociative disorder that may lead to homicide or suicide.

Susto or Espanto

Susto (Espanto) is seen in the High Andes. A prolonged depressive episode occurs that is believed to result from supernatural agencies.

Windigo or Wihtigo

Windigo (Wihtigo) is seen in North American Indian tribes. It is a depressive disorder in which patients believe they have mutated into cannibalistic monsters.

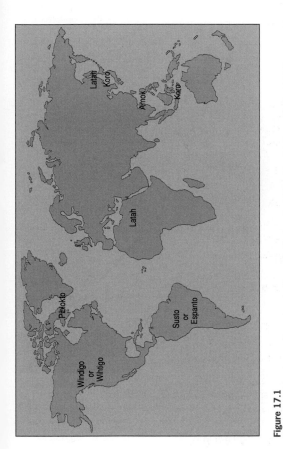

Figure 17.1
Culture-bound syndromes (Reproduced with permission from Puri BK, Laking PJ, Treasaden IH 1996 Textbook of psychiatry. Edinburgh: Churchill Livingstone.)

Forensic psychiatry

This chapter outlines aspects of civil law and criminal responsibility with which the psychiatrist may be involved and describes the main headings that need to be used in a psychiatric court report.

CIVIL LAW

Civil law deals with legislation concerning contracts, property and inheritance.

Testamentary capacity

This is the capacity to make a legally valid will. In order to do so, at the time of making the will the person doing so (the testator) should be of 'sound disposing mind' and:

- Understand what a will is
- Know the nature and extent of his or her property
- Know the names of those having a claim on his or her property, and be able to assess the relative merits of those claims
- Be free from an abnormal state of mind that might distort his or her feelings or judgements with respect to the will.

CRIMINAL RESPONSIBILITY
Fitness to plead

In order to be fit to plead under English law, a defendant should be able to:

- Understand the nature of the charge
- Understand the difference between pleading guilty and not guilty

- Instruct Counsel for the defence
- Challenge jurors
- Follow evidence in the court.

Mens rea

To be convicted of a crime, it must not only be proved that the defendant carried out the criminal act (*actus rea*), but also that he or she had a guilty state of mind at the material time (*mens rea*). The defence that the defendant did not have a necessary degree of *mens rea* may be made on the grounds of:

- Being not guilty by reason of insanity (the McNaughton Rules)
- Diminished responsibility (used when charged with murder, the defendant pleading not guilty of murder but guilty of manslaughter on the grounds of diminished responsibility)
- Being unable to form an intent owing to an automatism (an act over which the defendant had no control, e.g. sleepwalking).

PSYCHIATRIC COURT REPORT

This should contain the following information:

- The name, date of birth and address of the defendant
- Where and when the interview was carried out and who was present
- At whose request the interview was carried out
- Sources of information
- Family history
- Developmental history
- Psychosexual history
- Occupational history
- Personality
- Past medical and psychiatric history and current medication, if any
- Forensic history
- Drug and alcohol abuse
- Mental state at the time of the offence
- Current mental state

- Opinion, including fitness to plead
- Name, qualifications and appointment of the psychiatrist (and, in England and Wales, whether approved under Section 12 of the Mental Health Act 1983).

FINAL MEDICINE EXAMINATION: QUESTIONS AND ANSWERS

··

QUESTIONS
Chapter 1

1. Outline the headings of the psychiatric history.

2. Outline the headings of the mental state examination.

3. What first-line investigations would you perform on a patient with schizophrenia who has been readmitted to your ward with a relapse of his illness?

4. Outline the main headings you would use in giving an oral assessment of a psychiatric case in a clinical examination.

Chapter 2

1. What do the following terms mean?
   (a) Flight of ideas
   (b) Echolalia
   (c) Thought blocking
   (d) Neologism
   (e) Alexithymia
   (f) Dementia
   (g) Delusion.

2. What is the difference between mood and affect?

3. State Schneider's first-rank symptoms of schizophrenia.

4. How does an overvalued idea differ from a delusion?

5. Compare and contrast illusions, hallucinations and pseudohallucinations.

6. Give three examples of aphasias, explaining their definitions.

7. Give two ways in which the unconscious may be studied in psychoanalytic psychotherapy.

8. List five defence mechanisms.

Chapter 3

1. Outline the management of delirium.

2. Give four important causes of each of
   (a) Delirium
   (b) Dementia.

3. What is Korsakov's syndrome? Outline its aetiology, pathology and clinical features.

4. Compare and contrast the neuropsychiatric sequelae of damage to the frontal lobe and to the temporal lobe of the brain.

5. List five causes of an organic mood disorder.

Chapter 4

1. What is the difference between physical dependence and psychological dependence?

2. Define the terms dependence syndrome and tolerance.

3. What are the low-risk levels of alcohol consumption in men and women?

4. How many units of alcohol are contained in:
   (a) A pint of standard-strength beer
   (b) A standard measure of spirits
   (c) A glass of sherry
   (d) A bottle of spirits?

5. What are the clinical features of fetal alcohol syndrome?

6. How would you carry out a full assessment of a patient suspected of suffering from alcoholism?

7. What are the main features of 'cold turkey' and how can they be treated?

8. Compare and contrast the psychological actions of cannabis and cocaine.

9. List four withdrawal symptoms that may follow the abuse of amphetamines.

Chapter 5

1. Compare and contrast simple schizophrenia and paranoid schizophrenia.

2. What are the point prevalence and the lifetime risk of schizophrenia?

3. Why might schizophrenia be more common in those in social classes IV and V?

4. How would you treat a patient with acute (positive) schizophrenic symptoms?

5. What is meant by a delusional disorder?

6. Give four examples of delusional disorders, explaining briefly the nature of the delusion in each case.

Chapter 6

1. List the biological symptoms of depression.

2. In what ways does a depressive episode differ from bereavement?

3. Compare and contrast the treatment of mild depression with that of depressive stupor.

4. What are the clinical features of mania? What would you expect to find on examination of the mental state in this disorder?

5. How does hypomania differ from mania?

6. How would you treat a patient who presents with mania?

Chapter 7

1. In what ways does agoraphobia differ from social phobia?

2. Outline the management of panic disorder.

3. How would you manage the case of a patient who requires injections (for diabetes) but who has a needle phobia?

4. What are the clinical features of generalized anxiety disorder?

5. How would you treat a patient with an obsessive–compulsive disorder, in which she repeatedly engages in handwashing and cleaning rituals?

6. What is meant by a dissociative disorder? Give five examples of such a disorder.

Chapter 8

1. What are the main physical signs of anorexia nervosa?

2. Which psychiatric symptoms are most commonly associated with anorexia nervosa?

3. Which organic causes would you wish to exclude in a suspected case of anorexia nervosa?

4. Describe the management of anorexia nervosa.

5. What are the main physical signs of bulimia nervosa?

6. Describe the management of bulimia nervosa.

Chapter 9

1. Describe the main phases of the sexual response in both normal men and normal women.

2. What are the main causes of erectile dysfunction?

3. What are the main components of sex therapy, as devised by Masters and Johnson?

4. How might premature ejaculation be treated?

5. Compare and contrast transsexualism and dual-role transvestism.

6. What is meant by frotteurism?

Chapter 10

1. What do you understand by the term personality disorder?

2. Describe the key features of schizoid personality disorder.

3. Compare and contrast paranoid personality disorder with histrionic personality disorder.

4. What is meant by dependent personality disorder?

Chapter 11

1. What is the prevalence of psychiatric disorder in children?

2. What are the cardinal features of ADHD?

3. Outline the management of ADHD.

4. What is meant by a conduct disorder?

5. What are the clinical features of elective mutism?

6. Give the clinical features of enuresis.

7. Which organic disorders should be excluded in children with enuresis?

8. Describe the management of functional enuresis in children.

9. Give the clinical features of encopresis.

10. Describe the management of functional encopresis in children.

11. What do you understand by the term pica?

12. Describe the clinical features of tic disorders.

13. What are the main features of Asperger's syndrome?

Chapter 12

1. How can mental retardation be classified according to IQ?

2. What are the main clinical features of Down's syndrome?

3. What are the main clinical features of childhood autism?

4. What are the main clinical features of Fragile X syndrome?

Chapter 13

1. How may depression present in the elderly?

2. How might you try to differentiate between pseudodementia and depression in the elderly?

3. What is meant by the term paraphrenia?

4. Which drugs are used as cognitive enhancers in Alzheimer's disease?

Chapter 14

1. Outline what is known about the epidemiology of suicide.

2. How common is psychiatric disorder in those who commit suicide? What are the commonest such psychiatric disorders?

3. How would you assess a case of attempted suicide?

4. What is meant by the term parasuicide?

Chapter 15

1. What are the main clinical features of premenstrual syndrome?

2. How common are postnatal blues? How would you manage this disorder?

3. What is known about the epidemiology of puerperal psychosis?

4. Describe the management of puerperal psychosis.

5. Compare and contrast the clinical features of puerperal psychosis and postnatal depression.

Chapter 16

1. What are the main extrapyramidal side effects of typical antipsychotics and why do they arise?

2. How would you recognize a case of neuroleptic malignant syndrome?

3. What are the main side-effects of lithium salts? How would you recognize lithium toxicity?

4. Which investigations would you carry out in monitoring a patient taking regular
   (a) Lithium carbonate
   (b) Carbamazepine?

5. What are the main antimuscarinic side-effects of amitriptyline?

6. Compare and contrast the modes of action of the different classes of antidepressant.

7. List five foods that should be avoided by patients taking MAOIs. Why are they dangerous?

8. Which drugs should be avoided by patients taking MAOIs?

9. Why is a RIMA safer than a MAOI?

10. Describe the main features of the benzodiazepine withdrawal syndrome.

11. List the main uses and contraindications of ECT.

12. What is cognitive therapy?

13. What is meant by the following terms
    (a) Sheltered workshop
    (b) Sheltered accommodation
    (c) Rehabilitation
    (d) Occupational therapy?

14. Give five examples of treatments based on behaviour therapy.

Chapter 17

1. How may depression present atypically in non-western immigrants to the west?

2. What is meant by a culture-bound syndrome? List two examples.

Chapter 18

1. What is meant by testamentary capacity?

2. List the criteria used to determine fitness to plead.

....

ANSWERS
Chapter 1

1. The headings of the psychiatric history are:

- Reason for referral
- Complaints
- History of presenting illness
- Family history
- Family psychiatric history
- Personal history (childhood, education, occupational history, psychosexual history, children, current social situation)
- Past medical history
- Past psychiatric history
- Psychoactive substance use (alcohol, tobacco, illicit drug abuse)
- Forensic history
- Premorbid personality.

2. The headings of the mental state examination are:

- Appearance and behaviour (general appearance, facial appearance, posture, movements, social behaviour, rapport, psychodynamic aspects)
- Speech (rate, quantity, articulation, form)
- Mood (objective assessment, subjective assessment, affect, anxiety)
- Thought content (preoccupations, obsessions, phobias, suicidal thoughts, homicidal thoughts)

- Abnormal beliefs and interpretation of events (content, onset, degree of intensity, rigidity)
- Abnormal experiences
- Cognitive state (orientation, attention and concentration, immediate recall, registration, short-term memory, memory for recent events, long-term memory, general knowledge, intelligence)
- Insight.

3. The first-line investigations that would be performed might include:

(i) Obtaining further information
Important sources of information might include:

- Relatives
- The patient's general practitioner
- Other professionals involved in the case, such as the patient's social worker and community psychiatric nurse, psychologists and hostel nursing staff (if appropriate)
- The past psychiatric case-notes
- Any other medical case-notes.

(ii) Blood tests
Haematological, biochemical, endocrine and serological blood tests that might be appropriate include:

- Full blood count, e.g. for anaemia and infections
- Urea and electrolytes, e.g. for renal function
- Thyroid function tests, e.g. for thyroid abnormalities
- Liver function tests, e.g. for encephalopathy
- Vitamin B_{12} and folate levels, e.g. for dementia and vitamin B_{12} deficiency
- Syphilis serology, e.g. for general paralysis of the insane.

(iii) Urinary tests
A urinary drug screen should be carried out to check for covert psychoactive substance abuse.

4. The main headings are:

- History
- Mental state examination
- Physical examination

- Brief summary of the main problems and the relevant positive and negative findings
- Investigations to be performed (or already carried out)
- Diagnosis or differential diagnosis — giving the main points in favour of and against each diagnosis
- Aetiological factors
- Management
- Prognostic factors.

Chapter 2

1. (a) This is a disorder of the form of speech and refers to speech that consists of a stream of accelerated thoughts with abrupt changes from topic to topic and no central direction. The connections between thoughts may be based on chance relationships, verbal associations, e.g. alliteration and assonance, clang associations (using words with a similar sound), punning (using the same word with more than one meaning) and distracting stimuli.

(b) Echolalia is a disorder of the form of speech in which another person's speech is automatically imitated by the patient.

(c) This is a disorder of the form of speech, in which a sudden interruption in the train of thought occurs, leaving a 'blank', after which what was being said cannot be recalled.

(d) A neologism is a word that is newly made up, or an everyday word that is used in a special way.

(e) This refers to difficulty in being aware of or describing one's emotions.

(f) Dementia refers to a global organic impairment of intellectual functioning without impairment of consciousness.

(g) A delusion is a false personal belief based on incorrect inference about external reality and is firmly sustained in spite of what almost everyone else believes and in spite of what constitutes incontrovertible and obvious proof or evidence to the contrary. The belief is not one normally held by others of the same subculture.

2. Mood is a pervasive and sustained emotion that, in the extreme, markedly colours the person's perception of the world. In contrast, affect is a pattern of observable behaviours that is the expression of a subjectively experienced feeling state (emotion), and is variable over time, in response to changing emotional states.

3. These are:
- Auditory hallucinations — voices repeating thoughts out loud; voices discussing the subject in the third person; a running commentary
- Thought insertion
- Thought withdrawal
- Thought broadcasting
- Made feelings, impulses and actions
- Somatic passivity
- Delusional perception.

4. An overvalued idea differs from a delusion in that although both involve a belief that is demonstrably false and not one normally held by others of the same subculture, the intensity with which the belief is held is less in the case of an overvalued idea: in the case of an overvalued idea there is an unreasonable and sustained intense preoccupation but this is maintained with less than delusional intensity, whereas in the case of a delusion the belief is firmly sustained.

5. The key points to note are that:
- All three are forms of sensory deception
- An illusion is a false perception of a real external stimulus
- An hallucination is a false sensory perception occurring in the absence of a real external stimulus
- A pseudohallucination is a form of imagery arising in the subjective inner space of the mind and lacking the substantiality of normal perceptions.

6. Agnostic alexia — words can be seen but not read.

   Pure word deafness — words that are heard cannot be comprehended.

   Visual asymbolia — words can be transcribed but not read.

Nominal aphasia — difficulty in naming objects.

Central (syntactical) aphasia — difficulty in arranging words in their correct sequence.

Expressive (motor) aphasia — difficulty is experienced in expressing thoughts in words but comprehension remains.

Global aphasia — both receptive (difficulty in the comprehension of word meanings) and expressive aphasia (difficulty in the expression of thoughts in words while comprehension remains) are present at the same time.

Jargon aphasia — incoherent, meaningless, neologistic speech occurs.

(Give any three).

7. The unconscious can be studied in psychoanalytic psychotherapy using the following:

- Free association — the articulation, without censorship, of all thoughts that come to mind is encouraged.
- Freudian slips (parapraxes) — unconscious thoughts slip through when censorship is off-guard.
- Dreams analysis — dreams may be based on the subject's unconscious wishes; indeed, Freud referred to dreams as the royal road to the unconscious.

(Give any two).

8. Defence mechanisms include:

- Denial
- Displacement
- Introjection and identification
- Isolation
- Projection
- Projective identification
- Rationalization
- Reaction formation
- Regression
- Repression
- Sublimation
- Undoing.

(Give any five.)

Chapter 3

1. Carry out relevant investigations. Good, calming nursing care is essential, preferably in a quiet single room. Ensure an adequate fluid and electrolyte balance. Explain the condition to the patient. Encourage correct orientation by allowing the patient to know the time, placing a television in the room and allowing visitors. A low level of lighting should be used at night.

    If the patient is very agitated, anxious or frightened, oral or intramuscular haloperidol can be used; if there is hepatic failure, benzodiazepines can be given. Benzodiazepines can also be prescribed at night for their hypnotic action.

2. (a) Important causes of delirium include:

- Drug toxicity
- Industrial poisons
- Carbon monoxide poisoning
- Drug and alcohol withdrawal
- Encephalitis
- Meningitis
- Head injury
- Subarachnoid haemorrhage
- Space occupying lesions
- Epilepsy and postictal states
- Primary hypoadrenalism (Addison's disease)
- Cushing's syndrome
- Hyperinsulinism
- Hypothyroidism
- Hyperthyroidism
- Hypopituitarism
- Hypoparathyroidism
- Hyperparathyroidism
- Hepatic failure
- Renal failure
- Respiratory failure
- Cardiac failure
- Pancreatic failure
- Hypoxia
- Hypoglycaemia
- Fluid and electrolyte imbalance
- Carcinoid syndrome

- Porphyria
- Thiamine deficiency
- Nicotinic acid deficiency
- Folate deficiency
- Vitamin B_{12} deficiency
- Systemic infections
- Postoperative states.

    (Give any four.)

(b) Important causes of dementia include:

- Alzheimer's disease
- Vascular (multi-infarct) dementia
- Pick's disease
- Huntington's disease
- Creutzfeldt–Jakob disease
- Normal-pressure (intermittent) hydrocephalus.

    (Give any four.)

3. Korsakov's syndrome (amnesic syndrome) is a syndrome of prominent impairment of recent and remote memory with preservation of immediate recall in the absence of generalized cognitive impairment. Retrograde amnesia (inability to recall events before the onset of the disorder) and anterograde amnesia (poor memory for events taking place after the onset of the disorder) occur.

Aetiology. It can be caused by thiamine deficiency (owing to alcohol abuse, malabsorption, hyperemesis or starvation), intoxication with heavy metals or carbon monoxide, head injury, tumours affecting the third ventricle or hippocampal formation, bilateral hippocampal damage, subarachnoid haemorrhage, infections (HSV or TB meningitis), epilepsy, hypoxia, and Alzheimer's disease.

Pathology. One or both of the following are typically affected:

- the hypothalamic–diencephalic system
- the bilateral hippocampal region.

Clinical features. The anterograde amnesia is associated with an impaired ability to learn and disorientation for time. If the underlying pathology improves this can result in a lessening of the extent of the retrograde amnesia.

Confabulation is a common feature. Other cognitive functions are usually normal, as is perception.

4. The neuropsychiatric sequelae of damage to the frontal lobe and to the temporal lobe of the brain tend to be distinct, with little in common.

Following frontal lobe damage, personality changes may occur, including disinhibition, reduced social and ethical control, sexual indiscretions, errors of judgement, elevated mood, lack of concern for the feelings of others and irritability. These are related to prefrontal impairment, and in frontal lobe damage are associated with perseveration, utilization behaviour and palilalia. Other characteristic features of frontal lobe damage include impaired attention, concentration and initiative. Aspontaneity, slowed psychomotor activity, motor Jacksonian fits and urinary incontinence may also occur. Involvement of the motor cortex or deep projections may cause a contralateral spastic paresis or aphasia. Posterior dominant frontal lobe lesions may cause apraxia of the face and tongue, primary motor aphasia or motor agraphia. Orbital lesions may cause anosmia and ipsilateral optic atrophy.

In contrast, sensory aphasia, alexia and agraphia are associated with dominant temporal lobe lesions while non-dominant temporal lobe lesions may cause hemisomatognosia, prosopagnosia, visuospatial difficulties and impaired retention and learning of non-verbal patterned stimuli. Bilateral medial lesions may cause the amnesic syndrome. Other features of temporal lobe damage may include psychotic symptoms, epilepsy (*not* motor Jacksonian fits as in frontal lobe damage) and a contralateral homonymous upper quadrantic visual field defect.

5. Causes of an organic mood disorder include:

- Psychoactive substance use
- Treatment with corticosteroids
- Treatment with L-dopa
- Treatment with clonidine
- Treatment with methyldopa
- Treatment with reserpine

- Treatment with oestrogens
- Treatment with clomiphene
- Hypothyroidism
- Hyperthyroidism
- Primary hypoadrenalism (Addison's disease)
- Cushing's syndrome
- Hypoglycaemia
- Hyperparathyroidism
- Hypopituitarism
- Pernicious anaemia
- Systemic lupus erythematosus
- Neoplasia
- Infections
- Parkinson's disease
- Head injury.

(Give any five.)

Chapter 4

1. Physical dependence refers to an adaptive state in which intense physical disturbance occurs when the administration of a psychoactive substance is suspended; there is a desire to take the substance to avoid the physical symptoms of the withdrawal state. In the case of psychological dependence, on the other hand, a psychoactive substance produces a feeling of satisfaction and a psychological drive that requires periodic or continuous administration of the substance to produce pleasure or to avoid the psychological discomfort of its absence.

2. *Dependence syndrome.* The use of psychoactive substances has a higher priority than other behaviours that once had higher value. There is a desire, often strong and overpowering, to take the substance(s) on a continuous or periodic basis. Tolerance may or may not be present.

   Tolerance. The desired central nervous system effects of a psychoactive substance diminish with repeated use, so that increasing doses are needed to achieve the same effects.

3. The Royal College of Physicians has defined low-risk levels of consumption as up to 21 units of alcohol per week for men, and up to 14 units per week for non-pregnant women. This amount should not be consumed in one go, and alcohol should not be consumed every day, for these levels to apply. Abstinence is recommended for pregnant women.

4. (a) 2.
   (b) 1.
   (c) 1.
   (d) 30.

5. The clinical features include:

- Microcephaly
- Ocular hypertelorism
- Mild to moderate mental retardation
- Poor growth
- Increased neonatal mortality
- Stabismus
- Small nose
- Long upper lip with narrow vermilion border
- Pectus excavatum
- Cardiac murmurs (e.g. from atrial septal defect).

6. A full assessment would include the following.

History. Look in particular for evidence of difficulties at work (e.g. absenteeism and frequent changes of job) and high risk occupation, psychosexual and relationship difficulties, repeated accidents, withdrawal symptoms, a family history of alcohol problems, a forensic history (e.g. drink-driving offences). The alcohol history should include the pattern of drinking and the average number of units consumed weekly.

Screen with the CAGE Questionnaire:

- Have you ever felt you should *Cut down* on your drinking?
- Have people *Annoyed* you by criticizing your drinking?
- Have you ever felt *Guilty* about your drinking?
- Have you ever had a drink first thing in the morning (an *Eye-opener*) to steady your nerves or get rid of a hangover?

   (Two or more positive answers are indicative of problem drinking.)

Mental state examination. Look for evidence of the psychopathology associated with chronic heavy alcohol consumption.

Physical examination. Look for evidence of withdrawal symptoms, liver disease, accidents or fighting, and illicit drug abuse.

Investigations. Further information is required. The following may be raised:

- Mean corpuscular volume (MCV)
- γ-Glutamyltransferase (γGT)
- Aspartate transaminase (AST)
- Blood alcohol concentration (measured from a blood sample or via expired air)
- Plasma uric acid concentration.

7. The main features of 'cold turkey' include a history of abuse of a psychoactive substance (usually opioids such as heroin), and an intense craving for the psychoactive substance, nausea and vomiting, muscle aches and joint pains, lacrimation and rhinorrhoea, dilated pupils, piloerection, sweating, diarrhoea, yawning, body temperature changes, restlessness and insomnia, increased cardiac rate, and abdominal pains. Treatment includes detoxification with chlormethiazole, a benzodiazepine, or, in the case of dependency on heroin, methadone.

8. Both cannabis and cocaine can lead to psychological dependence. Both may cause euphoria, impaired judgement, and hallucinations. Tactile hallucinations (formication — the sensation of insects crawling under the skin) characteristically occur with cocaine use (the so-called 'cocaine bug') but are not a characteristic feature of cannabis use. Cannabis is more likely to lead to suspiciousness, which may develop into persecutory delusions, a feeling that time is being slowed, and social withdrawal; cocaine is more likely to lead to grandiosity and increased sexual interest.

9. Withdrawal symptoms that may follow the abuse of amphetamines include:

- Delirium
- Dysphoric mood
- Fatigue

- Sleep disturbance (insomnia or hypersomnia)
- Agitation.

  (Give any four.)

Chapter 5

1. Simple schizophrenia is characterized by an insidious onset of decline in functioning socially and at work or in education; negative symptoms develop without the occurrence beforehand of positive symptoms. In contrast, paranoid schizophrenia is dominated by the presence of paranoid symptoms, such as delusions and hallucinations (positive symptoms).

2. The point prevalence of schizophrenia is 0.5–1 per cent of the population. The lifetime risk is approximately one per cent.

3. A reason why schizophrenia is more common in those in social classes IV and V is the phenomenon of social drift, whereby patients drift downwards socially owing to the illness.

4. The treatment should include:

- Taking a full history
- Carrying out a mental state examination
- Carrying out a full physical examination
- Hospitalization
- Routine first-line investigations
- Pharmacotherapy with antipsychotic medication
- Making appropriate provisions of outpatient care following discharge from hospital, paying due attention to factors that might be important such as compliance with medication (e.g. consider depot antipsychotic medication if non-compliance is likely), outpatient appointments, and the need for community psychiatric nursing follow-up, social worker input, occupational therapy, and so on; a care plan is required.

5. The core feature of such a disorder is the development of a delusion or delusional system which is usually persistent, sometimes lifelong, and does not have an identifiable organic basis. Occasional or transitory auditory hallucinations, particularly in elderly patients, may occur.

6. Give any four of the following:

Capgras' syndrome. A person who is familiar to the patient is believed to have been replaced by a double. It is commoner in women, with the apparently replaced person often being a relative.

Cotard's syndrome. A nihilistic delusional disorder in which, for example, the patient believes their money, friends or body parts do not exist.

Erotomania (de Clérambault's syndrome). The patient holds the delusional belief that someone else, usually of a higher social or professional status, is in love with them. It is more common in women.

Fregoli's syndrome. The patient believes that a familiar person, who is often believed to be the patient's persecutor, has taken on different appearances.

Induced psychosis (folie à deux). Two (or more) people who are closely related emotionally share the delusional disorder. One has a genuine psychotic disorder and their delusional system is induced in the other, who may be dependent or less intelligent.

Pathological (delusional) jealously. The patient holds the delusional belief that his or her spouse or sexual partner is being unfaithful and goes to great lengths to find evidence of this. It is more common in men.

Persecutory (querulant) delusions. Patients suffer from a delusional system in which they believe they are being persecuted.

Chapter 6

1. These are:

- Decreased appetite
- Weight loss
- Constipation
- Sleep disturbance, such as early morning wakening, initial insomnia, or broken sleep
- Diurnal variation of mood
- Decreased libido
- Amenorrhoea.

2. The following are more likely to point to a depressive episode than bereavement:

- Guilt about things other than actions taken or not taken by the survivor at the time of death
- Thoughts of death other than the survivor feeling that he or she would be better off dead or should have died with the deceased
- Morbid preoccupation with worthlessness
- Marked psychomotor retardation
- Prolonged and marked functional impairment
- Hallucinations other than thinking that one hears the voice of, or transiently sees the image of, the deceased.

3. Mild depression can usually be treated on an outpatient basis, whereas hospitalization is essential in the case of depressive stupor. Mild depression can be treated with psychotherapy, for example cognitive behavioural therapy (CBT), and/or antidepressant medication in relatively low doses. In contrast, depressive stupor may require electroconvulsive therapy as a first-line treatment, and/or high dose antidepressant medication. The physical condition of the patient (e.g. fluid balance, urea and electrolyte levels, full blood count, etc.) must be monitored in the case of depressive stupor, but not usually in the case of mild depression.

4. In mania there is elevation of mood, increased energy, overactivity, pressure of speech, reduced sleep, loss of normal social and sexual inhibitions, and poor attention and concentration. The elevated mood may manifest itself as euphoria, but sometimes patients can instead be irritable and angry. The patient may overspend, start unrealistic projects, be sexually promiscuous, and, if irritable or angry, be inappropriately aggressive. Neglect of eating, drinking and personal hygiene may result in dangerous states of dehydration and self-neglect.

Mental state examination:

Appearance. The patient may be flamboyantly dressed. In severe cases signs of self-neglect may be present (e.g. appearing unkempt and dehydrated).

Behaviour. Overactivity is characteristic. The patient may not sit still.

Speech. There is pressure of speech. Flight of ideas is common in severe mania, with the connections between topics being based, for example, on chance relationships, verbal associations, clang associations, and distracting stimuli.

Mood. Euphoria or irritability occur.

Thought content and abnormal beliefs. The patient has an inflated view of his or her self-importance and has expansive and grandiose ideas about the significance of his or her opinions and work. These may develop into delusions. Irritability and suspiciousness may develop into delusions of persecution.

Abnormal experiences. Subjective hyperacusis and auditory or visual hallucinations may occur.

Cognition. Poor attention and concentration occur.

Insight. Insight is characteristically absent.

5. Hypomania is simply a lesser degree of mania.
6. A detailed history should be obtained (from the patient and appropriate informants), and a full mental state examination and physical examination must be carried out. The first-line investigations should be carried out (see Answer to Chapter 1, Question 3).

Hospitalization. The patient should be admitted, compulsorily if need be. If suffering from self-neglect and dehydration, these should be treated in addition to the manic symptoms.

Drug treatment. **Antipsychotic** drugs such as haloperidol and chlorpromazine (given intramuscularly if necessary) act rapidly and are the mainstay of the treatment of acute mania. **Lithium** salts (lithium carbonate and lithium citrate) are used in the prophylaxis of mania and, therefore, the patient should be started on lithium while an inpatient in order to prevent future relapses. Lithium has a low therapeutic ratio and therefore regular plasma level monitoring is essential to keep the plasma lithium concentration between 0.4 and 1.0 mmol l^{-1} (measured 12 hours after the last dose). Urea and electrolytes and thyroid function tests need to be monitored regularly while taking lithium. If the disorder is resistant to lithium, prophylactic **carbamazepine** can be tried, with regular plasma level monitoring.

Electroconvulsive therapy (ECT). This is used in treating rare cases of manic stupor.

Family therapy. This may be needed if the patient is subjected to a high level of expressed emotion.

Care plan. A detailed care plan should be devised before discharging the patient.

Chapter 7

1. In social phobia the phobias are centred around a fear of scrutiny by other people in comparatively small groups, as opposed to crowds in agoraphobia. Social phobia often begins in adolescence, whereas agoraphobia often starts later, in the 20s and 30s. Agoraphobia is more common in females, whereas the sex ratio is equal for social phobia.

2.

History and mental state examination. A history and mental state examination should be carried out, for example in order to rule out a depressive episode.

Physical examination and investigations. A physical examination and investigations should be carried out in order to exclude organic disorders such as hypoglycaemic episodes, hyperthyroidism and phaeochromocytoma.

Supportive measures. The patient should be reassured and the causes of individual symptoms, e.g. palpitations, should be given to allay unnecessary worry.

Drug treatment. Antidepressants (e.g. imipramine) are effective in treating panic disorder, whether or not there is an underlying depressive disorder. Anxiolytics, including buspirone and benzodiazepines, can be used for the short-term management of anxiety disorders.

Cognitive therapy. In patients worried about the physical consequences of anxiety symptoms, e.g. that palpitations are related to heart disease, the symptoms are induced voluntarily, e.g. by hyperventilation or exercise, and the nature of the symptoms is explained.

3. The treatment of choice is behaviour therapy, involving exposure combined with anxiety management.

4. The key clinical feature is the occurrence of generalized and persistent anxiety that is not restricted to, or even strongly predominating in, any particular environmental situation, that is, it is free-floating. Symptoms can result from sympathetic overactivity, increased muscle tension, and hyperventilation, and commonly include a continuous feeling of nervousness, trembling, muscular tension, sweating, cool clammy hands, light-headedness, tension headaches, palpitations, tachycardia, dizziness, dry mouth, dysphagia, breathlessness, flushes, fatigue, epigastric discomfort, and increased frequency and urgency of micturition. Sleep disturbance may occur, typically with initial insomnia while the patient lies in bed worrying, and broken sleep thereafter.

5. Take a full history and carry out a mental state examination; in addition to confirming the diagnosis, this may reveal any coexisting or underlying depressive disorder. If such a depressive disorder is found, it should be treated. The treatment of the obsessive–compulsive disorder should include supportive measures, in which the patient is reassured that she is not 'mad', and the disorder and treatment plan should be carefully explained. If the patient carries out her compulsions as a result of a fear of dirt, then behaviour therapy can be attempted, in which she is exposed to the 'dirty' objects and not then allowed immediately to engage in handwashing or cleaning rituals (response prevention). If this is not effective, then pharmacotherapy with a selective serotonin reuptake inhibitor may be tried; the patient should be told about the side-effects to be expected from such treatment.

6. This is a disorder in which there is a partial or complete loss of the normal integration between memories of the past, awareness of identity and immediate sensations, and control of bodily movements, which is psychogenic in origin, being closely associated in time with traumatic events, insoluble and intolerable problems, or disturbed relationships. Examples include:

- Dissociative amnesia
- Dissociative fugue
- Dissociative stupor
- Trance and possession disorders
- Dissociative disorders of movement and sensation
- Ganser's syndrome
- Multiple personality disorder.

  (Give any five.)

Chapter 8

1. Physical signs may include:

- Cachexia
- Muscle wasting with good power
- Dehydration
- Salivary gland swelling
- Dental caries and perimyolysis
- Lanugo hair is often present on the face and back
- Axillary and pubic hair are present (if post pubertal)
- Poor peripheral circulation
- Anaemia
- Cardiovascular abnormalities, including arrhythmias, bradycardia, hypotension, oedema.

2. The psychiatric symptoms most commonly associated with anorexia nervosa are:

- *Obsessive–compulsive behaviour*, e.g. compulsive handwashing and weight checking.
- *Anxiety*, particularly related to food and eating.
- *Mood disorder*, including depressive episodes (with suicidal thoughts, poor concentration and social withdrawal) and labile mood.

3. These include:

- Chronic debilitating diseases
- Brain tumours
- Intestinal disorders such as Crohn's disease or malabsorption syndromes.

4. A full history should be taken and mental state examination carried out, in order to establish the diagnosis and exclude other psychiatric disorders (see

Answer to Chapter 8, Question 2). A physical examination (including body mass and height) and first-line investigations should be carried out in order to establish the body mass index, the degree of any complications, and to help exclude organic causes of weight loss (see Answer to Chapter 8, Question 3). The condition should be explained to the patient and her or his family. The need for controlled weight gain should be agreed with the patient in the context of a therapeutic relationship.

Hospitalization. This is required if there is:

- Severe weight loss
- A high rate of loss of weight
- Severe metabolic disturbance or infection
- A severe depressive episode or risk of suicide
- Failure to maintain weight gain agreed in an outpatient contract
- A family crisis.

The admission should ideally be planned and mutually agreed, but if voluntary admission is refused and there is danger to life, compulsory admission should be considered.

Inpatient treatment. This includes:

- Keeping weight and fluid charts
- Controlled refeeding
- A behavioural regime may be used, e.g. starting with bed rest which is gradually relaxed as weight is gained at a previously agreed rate
- Psychotherapy, initially supportive psychotherapy followed by cognitive and family therapies (see below) as progress is made.

Outpatient treatment.

- Supportive psychotherapy helps to contain the difficulties encountered by the patient while she or he is aided in the process of keeping to an agreed diet, encouraged not to lose weight and assisted in developing better interpersonal relationships.
- Cognitive therapy aims to identify and change inappropriate cognitions regarding eating behaviour,

except the genital areas (sensate focus stage). In the next stage they are encouraged to give pleasure without engaging in intercourse; communication with the partner is relied on and mutual masturbation allowed. Finally, full sexual intercourse is permitted.

4. The squeeze technique or the stop–start method can be used. Both are usually introduced at the genital sensate focus stage of sex therapy (see previous Answer). In both techniques, the partner strokes the penis to a point of high arousal before ejaculatory inevitability occurs. In the squeeze technique, the glans penis is then squeezed in order to delay ejaculation, while in the stop–start method the arousal is allowed to subside by cessation of the caressing. The cycle is repeated several times before finally masturbating the man to ejaculation. The techniques are based on the premise that premature ejaculation occurs because of excessively rapid male arousal and a lack of identification of the point of ejaculatory inevitability.

5. Both transsexualism and dual-role transvestism are gender identity disorders and both involve cross-dressing. However, while in transsexualism there is a desire to live and be accepted as a member of the opposite sex (usually accompanied by a sense of discomfort with one's anatomical sex and a wish to have treatment (hormonal and surgical) to make one's body as congruent as possible with the preferred sex), in dualrole transvestism there is no wish to become a member of the opposite sex.

6. Frotteurism is a disorder of sexual preference in which touching and rubbing against a non-consenting person is a sexually arousing stimulus.

Chapter 10

1. Personality disorders are deeply ingrained and enduring behaviour patterns manifesting as inflexible responses to a broad range of personal and social situations. They represent extreme or significant deviations from the way average individuals in a given culture perceive, think, feel and relate to others. They

are often associated with subjective distress and problems in social functioning and performance. They tend to appear in late childhood or adolescence and continue to be manifest into adulthood: therefore, it is unlikely that a diagnosis of personality disorder is appropriate below the age of 17 years.

2. There is an indifference to social relationships and a restricted range of emotional expreience and expression. Few, if any, activities give pleasure and individuals tend to be emotionally cold, detached or flat with a limited ability to express feelings of warmth or anger towards others. Solitary activities are preferred and there is a preoccupatin with fantasy and introspection.

3. An important feature of paranoid personality disorder is a tendency to interpret the actions of others as being deliberately demeaning or threatening. In contrast, in histrionic personality disorder there is excessive emotionality and attention-seeking, with self-dramatization, theatricality, suggestibility, shallow and labile affectivity, and over-concern with physical attractiveness. While paranoid personality disorder is characteristically associated with an excessive sensitivity to setbacks and a tendency to bear grudges, be suspicious, and to be preoccupied with unsubstantiated conspiratorial explanations of events, in histrionic personality disorder excitement is continually sought, as is the appreciation of others and activities that allow one to be the centre of attention.

4. This is a personality disorder in which there is characteristically a tendency to dependent and submissive behaviour in which others are encouraged or allowed to make the patient's important decisions and the patient is unwilling to make any demands on people on whom he or she depends. Being alone feels uncomfortable owing to feelings of helplessness and there is difficulty in initiating projects.

Chapter 11

1. A study (by Rutter and colleagues) of 10- and 11-year-olds in the Isle of Wight in 1970 found that the one-year prevalence of psychiatric disorder was 6.8%, with the

rate in boys being twice that in girls. Of the 6.8%, 3% had conduct disorder and 2% emotional disorder. The prevalence increased with reduced IQ and there was a strong association with physical handicap and particularly with brain injury. A similar survey in an inner London borough, in which there was a high prevalence of overcrowding, found that the one-year prevalence of psychiatric disorder was 13%, about double that in the Isle of Wight.

2. The core features consist of the cluster of age-inappropriate behavioural abnormalities of the triad

- Inattention
- Hyperactivity
- Impulsivity.

There is impaired attention and overactivity, and both occur in more than one situation, e.g. at home, in school, at a clinic. Impaired attention leads to frequent changes from one activity to another and unfinished activities. Overactivity manifests as excessive restlessness e.g. running and jumping around, noisiness, and excessive talkativeness. Associated features include disinhibition in social relationships, recklessness and the impulsive defying of rules. These behaviour problems should start before the age of 6 years and be of long duration for an ICD-10 diagnosis of hyperkinetic disorder; symptoms of inattention, hyperactivity and impulsivity should have persisted for at least six months to a degree that is maladaptive and inconsistent with the developmental level for a DSM-IV diagnosis of ADHD.

3. A full child psychiatric interview should be carried out (see Table 11.2).

Support and advice. For parents and teachers.

Remedial teaching.

Behaviour modification. Appropriate methods can be taught to parents and teachers to prevent reinforcement of problem behaviour.

Drug treatment. Under specialist supervision, central nervous system stimulants (amphetamines and pemoline) can be used. Such use must be selective owing to side-effects such as irritability, depressed mood, insomnia, reduced appetite, and retarded growth.

4. The characteristic features of this disorder are a repetitive and persistent pattern of dissocial, aggressive or defiant conduct, which at its most extreme amounts to major violations of age-appropriate social expectations and is therefore more severe than ordinary childish mischief or adolescent rebelliousness. An isolated dissocial or criminal act is not sufficient to make this diagnosis, for which an enduring pattern of dissocial behaviour is required.

5. There is characteristically a marked, emotionally determined selectivity in speaking, such that the child demonstrates language competence in some situations but fails to speak in other (definable) situations. The failure to speak is not caused by a lack of knowledge of, or comfort with, the spoken language required in the social situation. The disturbance is not better accounted for by a communication disorder (e.g. stuttering) and does not occur exclusively during the course of a pervasive developmental disorder, schizophrenia, or other psychotic disorder.

   The disorder usually first manifests in early childhood, has a prevalence of about one in 1000 children, and affects males and females equally.

6. Functional (non-organic) enuresis is the involuntary passage of urine, by day and/or by night, which is abnormal in relation to the individual's mental age and which is not the result of a physical disorder. Nocturnal (bedwetting) enuresis occurs in about 10% of 5-year-olds, 5% of 10-year-olds, and 1% of 15-year-olds; the prevalence of diurnal (daytime) enuresis is lower. Nocturnal enuresis is commoner is boys, and diurnal enuresis in girls.

7. The following organic disorders should be excluded;

- Urinary tract infection
- Diabetes mellitus
- Neurological disorders - particularly epilepsy
- Structural abnormality of the urinary tract.

8. *Assessment.* A full child psychiatric interview should be carried out (see Table 11.2) in order to confirm the

diagnosis and exclude both physical causes (see previous Answer) and psychiatric causes.

Fluid intake. Parents should be advised to limit the child's intake of fluid before bedtime in the case of functional nocturnal enuresis.

Star chart. The child can be rewarded with stars on a chart for keeping dry.

Bell-and-pad. If the above measures do not help, a buzzer or bell-and-pad method, in which a bell sounds when urine is passed and wets a pad under the sheets, is used. This can be combined with the star chart method.

Drug treatment. A small dose of a tricyclic antidepressant will usually stop enuresis, owing to its antimuscarinic action. However, disadvantages include a high relapse rate, side-effects and the toxicity risk in accidental or intentional overdose (e.g. by siblings).

9. Functional (non-organic) encopresis is the repeated voluntary or involuntary passage of faeces, usually of normal or near-normal consistency, in appropriate places after an age at which bowel control is usual, in the absence of an organic cause. Faecal incontinence occurs at least once per week in 6% of 3-year-olds and 1.5% of 7-year-olds. It is three to four times commoner in boys than girls.

10. *Assessment.* A full child psychiatric interview should be carried out (see Table 11.2) in order to confirm the diagnosis and exclude physical causes such as chronic constipation and in order to assess emotional factors.

Behavioural. A programme in which the child is rewarded (e.g. using a star chart) for sucessfully passing faeces following each meal may prove successful.

Psychotherapy. Individual psychotherapy and family therapy may be required if there are emotional difficulties and/or problems with the relationship between the child and parent(s).

Drug treatment. Microenemata, smooth muscle stimulants, stool softeners, bulk agents and suppositories may be variously required (e.g. in retention).

11. This is the persistent eating of substances normally considered inedible, e.g. soil, paint chippings, and paper.

12. There is some form of tic, that is, rapid, involuntary, recurrent, non-rhythmic motor movement or vocal production of sudden onset and with no apparent purpose. In Gilles de la Tourette syndrome complex tics, involving the limbs and trunk, occur together with the echolalia, echopraxia, coprolalia, and copropraxia. Ten to 20% of children show transient tics at some time. Gilles de la Tourette syndrome is rare, occurring in approximately four to five individuals per 10000, and can occur in adults as well as in children and adolescents. Tic disorders are commoner in males: for Gilles de la Tourette syndrome, the male to female ratio is approximately 1.5:1 to 3:1.

13. This is a disorder characterized by the same kind of abnormalities of social interaction that occur in autism, together with a restricted, stereotyped, repetitive repertoire of interests and activities, but that differs from autism primarily in that there is no general delay or retardation in language or in cognitive development. The abnormalities of social interaction may include: a marked impairment in the use of multiple nonverbal behaviours such as eye-to-eye gaze, facial expression, body postures, and gestures to regulate social interaction; failure to develop peer relationships appropriate to development level; a lack of spontaneous seeking to share enjoyment, interests, or achievements with others (e.g. by a lack of showing, bringing, or pointing out objects of interest to other people); and a lack of social or emotional reciprocity. Psychotic episodes may occur in early adult life. The disorder is six to eight times more common in boys than in girls.

Chapter 12

1. Based on IQ, ICD-10 classifies mental retardation into the following groups:

- Mild mental retardation: IQ 50 to 69 (inclusive)
- Moderate mental retardation: IQ 35 to 49 (inclusive)
- Severe mental retardation: IQ 20 to 34 (inclusive)
- Profound mental retardation: IQ under 20.

2. Down's syndrome is a common cause of mental retardation, with an incidence of between one in 600 and one in 700 live births. 95% of cases result from trisomy 21 following non-disjunction during meiosis, 4 % are caused by translocation involving chromosome 21, while the remainder are mosaics. The majority of Down's syndrome babies are born to mothers aged over 35 years. Down's syndrome is characterized by learning disability (the intelligence quotient is usually below 70), bradycephaly, widely spaced eyes with epicanthic folds and oblique palpebral fissures, Brushfield spots, a small nose and mouth, a horizontally furrowed tongue, a high arched palate, malformed ears, broadening and shortening of the neck and hands, a single transverse palmar crease, curvature of the fifth finger, increased range of joint movements, stunted growth, and hypotonia. It is associated with an increased incidence of cataracts, epilepsy, specific auditory discrimination difficulties, congenital cardiac disease, umbilical herniae, oesophageal and duodenal atresia, respiratory infections and acute leukaemia.

3. Childhood autism is characterized by a general and profound failure to develop social relationship (autistic aloneness), speech and language retardation, ritualistic and compulsive behaviour, and an onset before the age of 30 months. Common features include poor eye contact, a lack of socioemotional reciprocity, echolalia, palilalia, a lack of social usage of language, a relative lack of creativity and fantasy in thoughts, increased self-injury (e.g. wrist biting) and stereotyped behaviour such as hand-flapping, nodding and rocking. There is a resistance to change in routine. Odd attachments to unusual objects may occur. There is an increased risk of epilepsy during adolescence. The disorder has a prevalence of two per 10000 children in the community. When those with severe mental retardation are included, the prevalence is increased. Autism can occur in association with all levels of intelligence, but significant learning disability (mental retardation) occurs in about 75% of cases of autism.

4. Fragile X syndrome is commoner in males, affecting 0.1% of males, it is particularly associated with large floppy ears, prognathism and macro-orchidism;

learning disability, joint hyperextensibility, soft velvety skin, a single palmer crease, flat feet, mitral valve prolapse, blue eyes and a large forehead are also more common. Female carriers have an increased likelihood of having poor muscular tone, joint hyperextensibility, prominent ears and elongated faces; one-third has reduced intellectual functioning.

Chaper 13

1. Depression may present typically or atypically. [For the typical presentation, give the clinical features described in Chapter 6, including the biological symptoms in the Answer to Question 1 of that chapter.] Atypical presentations may include:

   Depressed elderly patients may present atypically with:

- Agitated depression
- Symptoms masked by concurrent physical illness
- Minimization or denial of low mood
- Hypochondriasis
- Complaints of loneliness
- Complaints disproportionate to organic pathology and pain of unknown origin
- Onset of neurotic symptoms
- Depressive pseudodementia
- Behavioural disturbance (e.g. food refusal, aggressive behaviour, shoplifting, alcohol abuse)

2. You should base your answer on Table 13.1.
3. In ICD-10 'paraphrenia (late)' is included within 'delusional disorder'. Paraphrenia (delusional disorder) in the elderly is particularly likely to occur in those who live alone and have sensory deprivation, e.g. from poor eyesight or hearing difficulties. An elderly patient presenting with paraphrenia should therefore have their eyesight and hearing checked.
4. At the time of writing the following two reversible acetylcholinesterase inhibitors may be prescribed in Britain as cognitive enhancers in Alzheimer's disease:

- Donepezil
- Rivastigmine.

Chapter 14

1. *Sex ratio.* Commoner in males.

   Age. Commoner in those aged over 45 years.

   Marriage. Highest rates in those who are divorced, single or widowed. Those who are married have the lowest rate.
   Social class. Highest rates in social classes I and V.

   Employment. Associated with lack of employment, including both unemployment and retirement.

   Season. Highest rates in spring and early summer.

2. Psychiatric disorder is present in 90 per cent of those who commit suicide. The commonest such psychiatric disorders are:

- Depressive episodes
- Alcohol dependence
- Illicit drug abuse
- Personality disorder
- Chronic neuroses
- Schizophrenia.

3. In a case of attempted suicide it is important to determine the degree of suicidal intent that existed at the time of the attempt and that currently exists. Questions that should be answered include:

- What is the explanation for the attempt in terms of the likely reason(s) and goal(s)?
- What was the reaction of the patient to the fact that he or she failed to die?
- Does the patient intend to die now?
- Was the attempt planned beforehand, and if so, to what extent?
- Were any precautions taken to avoid discovery (such as locking the door and not expecting any visitors)?
- What method was used?
- Before the attempt, was there a final act such as making a will or leaving a suicide note?
- What problems confront the patient?
- Is there a psychiatric disorder and, if so, how relevant is it to the attempt?

- What are the patient's coping resources and supports?
- What kind of help might be appropriate, and is the patient willing to accept such help?

A high degree of suicidal intent is indicated by the following:

- Planning beforehand
- Precautions taken to avoid discovery
- No attempt made to seek help afterwards
- A dangerous method was used, e.g. shooting, drowning, hanging or electrocution
- There was a final act
- Extensive premeditation
- Admission of suicidal intent.

4. The term parasuicide refers to any self-initiated act deliberately undertaken by a patient who mimics the act of suicide, but which does not result in a fatal outcome. It is an act in which the patient injures himself or herself or takes a substance in a quantity which exceeds the therapeutic dose (if any) of his or her habitual level of consumption, and which he or she believes to be pharmacologically active.

Chapter 15

1. In preminstrual syndrome, psychological and physical symptoms recur, starting during the time between ovulation and menstruation, and ending soon after the onset of menstruation. Psychological symptoms include:

- Irritability
- Anxiety
- Tension
- Tiredness
- Depressed mood.

Common physical symptoms and signs of premenstrual syndrome include:

- Headache
- Acne
- Weight gain
- Breast tenderness and swelling

- Backache
- Stomach cramps
- A bloated feeling
- Swollen fingers and ankles.

Premenstrual syndrome occurs in 30–80 per cent of menstruating women.

2. Postnatal blues occur in over 50 per cent of mothers. The management includes an assessment (history and mental state examination) to establish the diagnosis and exclude any other diagnoses. Reassurance and explanation is usually all that is needed, as the condition is short-lived.

3. It occurs in about one in 500 live births with an onset usually between day 3. and day 14 postpartum. It is commoner in primigravidae. There are three subtypes, with the following relative prevalence rates in the West:

- Affective: 70 to 80 per cent (of cases of puerperal psychosis)
- Schizophrenic: 20 to 25 per cent
- Organic psychoses: very rare.

4. A full assessment should include a history, mental state examination and physical examination. Having established the diagnosis, hospitalization is usually required, preferably in a mother and baby unit so that the baby can be cared for by the nursing staff when the mother is too ill, and by the mother when she is better. The close proximity of the baby to his or her mother helps encourage bonding and diminishes feelings of guilt in the mother. The treatment is that which is standard for the type of puerperal psychosis present (i.e. that for a mood disorder or for schizophrenia). If a drug given to the mother is excreted in significant amounts in breast milk, then breast-feeding may have to be stopped. Electroconvulsive therapy (ECT) may need to be given in cases of severe depression because of its rapid action, so allowing the mother to resume caring for her baby sooner.

5. Puerperal psychosis may be affective or schizophrenic (or very rarely these days, in the West, organic) in its presentation, whereas postnatal depression always presents with depressive symptoms While puerperal

psychosis occurs in about one in 500 live births, postnatal depression is much more common, occurring in 10–15 per cent of mothers. The onset of puerperal psychosis is usually between day 3 and day 14 postpartum, whereas the onset of postnatal depression is generally later, usually two to six weeks postpartum. While puerperal psychosis is commoner in primigravidae, there is no association between previous pregnancies and the occurrence of postnatal depression.

Chapter 16

1. The main extrapyramidal side-effects of typical antipsychotics are:

- Parkinsonism
- Dystonias
- Akathisia
- Tardive dyskinesia.

They arise as a result of the antidopaminergic action of typical antipsychotics on the nigrostriatal system of the brain.

2. This is rare but potentially fatal toxic delirious state that may occur in patients taking certain psychotropic medications (such as chlorpromazine). It is characterized by:

- Hyperthermia
- A fluctuating level of consciousness
- Muscular rigidity
- Autonomic dysfunction (tachycardia, labile blood pressure, pallor, sweating and urinary incontinence).

Abnormal investigation results include:

- Increased creatinine phosphokinase
- Increased white blood count
- Abnormal liver function tests.

3. The main side-effects of lithium salts are:

- Gastrointestinal side-effects — nausea, vomiting and diarrhoea
- Fine tremor
- Dry mouth

- Polyuria
- Polydipsia
- Weight gain
- Oedema.

  Signs of lithium toxicity include:

- Blurred vision
- Increasing gastrointestinal disturbances — anorexia, vomiting and diarrhoea
- Muscle weakness
- Increased central nervous system disturbances — mild drowsiness and sluggishness increasing to giddiness with ataxia, coarse tremor, lack of coordination, and dysarthria.

(The presence of these signs requires immediate withdrawal of lithium treatment, to prevent severe over-dosage, associated with hyperreflexia and hyperextension of limbs, toxic psychoses, convulsions, syncope, oliguria, circulatory failure, coma and death.)

4. (a) The following blood tests should be carried out in monitoring a patient taking regular lithium carbonate:

- Plasma lithium level
- Urea
- Electrolytes
- Creatinine
- Thyroid function tests.

(The renal function should be checked before starting treatment with lithium carbonate.)

(b) The following blood tests should be carried out in monitoring a patient taking regular carbamazepine:

- Plasma carbamazepine level
- Full blood count.

(The full blood count and liver function tests should be checked before starting treatment with carbamazepine.)

5. These are:

- Dry mouth
- Blurred vision
- Constipation

- Urinary retention
- Sedation
- Nausea.

6. The essential points are:

- The antidepressant action of tricyclic antidepressants results from inhibiting the re-uptake of the monoamines noradrenaline and serotonin (5-HT).
- The antidepressant action of selective serotonin re-uptake inhibitors (SSRIs) results from selective central inhibition of the re-uptake of serotonin.
- The antidepressant action of selective noradrenaline and serotonin re-uptake inhibitors (SNRIs) results from selective central inhibition of the re-uptake of noradrenaline and serotonin.
- The antidepressant action of selective noradrenaline re-uptake inhibitors (NARIs) results from selective central inhibition of the re-uptake of noradrenaline.
- The antidepressant action of noradrenergic and specific serotonergic antidepressants (NaSSAs) results from the following actions. Central noradrenaline release is increased by antagonizing inhibitory presynaptic α_2-adrenoceptors. Serotonin release is increased by enhancing a facilitatory noradrenergic input to serotonergic cell bodies and by antagonizing inhibitory presynaptic α_2-adrenoceptors on serotonergic neuronal terminals.
- The antidepressant action of monoamine oxidase inhibitors (MAOIs) results from inhibiting the metabolic degradation of monoamines by the enzyme monoamine oxidase.
- The antidepressant action of reversible inhibitors of monoamine oxidase-A (RIMAs) results from the selective and reversible inhibition of the metabolic degradation of monoamines by monoamine oxidase type A (MAO-A).

7. Foods that should be avoided by patients taking MAOIs include:

- Cheese (*except* cottage cheese and cream cheese)
- Meat extracts and yeast extracts (e.g. Bovril, Marmite, Oxo)

- Alcohol (particularly Chianti, fortified wines and beer)
- Herring (pickled or smoked)
- Non-fresh fish, meat or poultry (e.g. seasoned game)
- Offal
- Avocado
- Banana skins
- Broad bean pods
- Caviar.

(Give any five.)

These foods are dangerous because they contain appreciable levels of tyramine. MAOIs interact dangerously with tyramine-containing foods by inhibiting the peripheral metabolism of pressor amines. Dietary tyramine can lead to a hypertensive crisis ('cheese reaction') in patients being treated with MAOIs.

8. Drugs that should be avoided by patients taking MAOIs include:

- Indirectly acting sympathomimetic amines (e.g. those found in cough mixtures and nasal decongestants)
- Tricyclic antidepressants
- Selective serotonin re-uptake inhibitors (SSRIs)
- Selective noradrenaline and serotonin re-uptake inhibitors (SNRIs)
- Selective noradrenaline re-uptake inhibitors (NARIs)
- Noradrenergic and specific serotonergic antidepressants (NaSSAs).

9. Since they are reversible, RIMAs can be displaced by other substances, such as tyramine, and therefore are much less likely to cause a food or drug interaction than are MAOIs.

10. If benzodiazepines are taken regularly for at least four weeks dependence may develop. When such regular intake is stopped suddenly, the benzodiazepine withdrawal syndrome occurs, which may include:

- Insomnia
- Anxiety symptoms
- Low mood
- Depersonalization
- Derealization

- Distorted perception of space
- Tinnitus
- Formication
- Influenza-like symptoms
- Loss of appetite and weight
- Seizures
- Confusional states
- Psychotic episodes.

11. The main uses of ECT are the treatment, in cases in which drug treatment is too slow or the patient resistant to drugs, of:

- Severe depressive illness (e.g. When there is a high immediate risk of suicide or insufficient fluid intake to maintain renal function)
- Puerperal depressive illness
- Mania
- Catatonic schizophrenia
- Schizoaffective disorder.

The main contraindications of ECT are:

- Physical disorders that may be worsened by the blood pressure rise caused by ECT, e.g. raised intracranial, cerebral aneurysm, recent myocardial infarction, cardiac arrhythmia
- Physical disorders that make anaesthesia risky, e.g. cardiac disease, chest infection.

12. Cognitive therapy is based on a model in which the processing of information is held to be of central importance and it is attempted to change this when treating psychiatric disorders. Disorders that have been found to respond include depression, phobic disorders, anxiety disorders and bulimia nervosa. Maladaptive thoughts are elicited and challenged during therapy. Examples seen in depression include:

- Arbitrary inference
- Catastrophizing
- Dichotomous thinking
- Maximization
- Minimization
- Overgeneralization

- Personalization
- Selective abstraction.

13. (a) This is a specially set up subsidised place of employment where the chronically ill (e.g. those with chronic schizophrenia) can obtain work experience and an increased sense of self-worth, if they cannot gain meaningful employment in the open market.

(b) This is a specially set up subsidised place of residence where the chronically ill (e.g. those with chronic schizophrenia) can live outside hospital, if they cannot cope with living on their own in the community. A hostel may be run by psychiatrically qualified staff, allowing the mental state, physical health and medication of the resident to be monitored.

(c) Rehabilitation programmes are used in treating chronically ill patients (e.g. those with chronic schizophrenia) who find it difficult to live outside hospital. A detailed assessment of disabilities and potential abilities is followed by setting goals and designing a plan to reach them. The programme is modified as required according to the response.

(d) This refers to a form of therapy in which a patient or hostel resident is taught skills required for daily living (e.g. shopping, cooking, and organizing one's life better) which may have been lost (e.g. in chronic schizophrenia) or never developed (e.g. in learning disabilities).

14. *Systematic desensitization.* Graded exposure, in reality or in imagination, takes place in conjunction with relaxation training. It can be used to treat phobic disorders.

Flooding. The patient is subjected to the stimulus all at once, and this is repeated until there is no longer any anxiety. It can be used to treat phobic disorders.

Response prevention. In treating obsessive–compulsive disorder, carrying out rituals is repeatedly prevented and the corresponding distress gradually diminishes.

Modelling. The patient physically follows the example of the therapist. It can be used to treat phobic disorders and compulsive rituals (e.g. concerning contamination).

Thought stopping. Unwanted thoughts are interrupted by thinking or saying aloud 'STOP' whenever the unwanted thought occurs; at first a rubber band worn around the wrist can also be snapped against the wrist when the unwanted thought occurs. It can be used to treat obsessional thoughts.

Assertiveness training. Roles are acted out in imaginary situations replicating circumstances found difficult in real life, using role-playing, role-reversal, modelling and coaching. It can be used to treat social phobia and shyness.

Social skills training. Role-playing, role-reversal, modelling, coaching and video feedback can be used to treat those with poor social skills.

Token economy. A system based on operant conditioning in which tokens given to reward desired behaviours become a secondary reinforcer (the tokens can be exchanged for goods or privileges). It can be used to alter the behaviour of long-stay patients and hostel residents with chronic schizophrenia or learning disability.

Pad-and-bell method. This can be used to treat nocturnal enuresis. A bell rings when bedwetting starts and the child has to get up and use the lavatory; in time, the bedwetting may stop.

Aversion therapy. Negative reinforcement is used to prevent unsuitable thoughts or behaviour. It is now rarely used.

(Give any five.)

Chapter 17

1. Depressed non-Western immigrants to the West may not complain of depression. Afro-Caribbean men may complain instead of erectile dysfunction or reduced libido while men and women from the Indian subcontinent may complain of somatic symptoms such as abdominal pains.
2. Culture-bound syndromes are specific disorders occurring in certain non-Western countries. Examples include:

- Amok

- Koro
- Latah
- Piblokto
- Susto or Espanto
- Windigo or Wihtigo.

   (Give any two.)

Chapter 18

1. Testamentary capacity is the capacity to make a legally valid will. In order to do so, at the time of making the will the person doing so (the testator) should be of 'sound disposing mind' and:

- Understand what a will is
- Know the nature and extent of his or her property
- Know the names of those having a claim on his or her property and be able to assess the relative merits of their claims
- Be free from an abnormal state of mind that might distort his or her feelings or judgements with respect to the will.

2. In order to be fit to plead under English law, a defendant should be able to:

- Understand the nature of the charge
- Understand the difference between pleading guilty and not guilty
- Instruct counsel for the defence
- Challenge jurors
- Follow evidence in the court.

Appendix I:
Mental Health
Legislation

This appendix briefly covers aspects of the Mental Health Act 1983, which applies in England and Wales. In Scotland the corresponding legislation is the Mental Health (Scotland) Act 1984, whereas in Northern Ireland it is the Mental Health (Northern Ireland) Order 1986.

SECTION 1: DEFINITIONS

Mental disorder
Mental illness, arrested or incomplete development of mind, psychopathic disorder and any other disorder or disability of mind.

Severe mental impairment
A state of arrested or incomplete development of mind which includes severe impairment of intelligence and social functioning, and is associated with abnormally aggressive or seriously irresponsible conduct on the part of the person concerned.

Mental impairment
A state of arrested or incomplete development of mind (not amounting to severe mental impairment) which includes significant impairment of intelligence and social functioning, and is associated with abnormally aggressive or seriously irresponsible conduct on the part of the person concerned.

Psychopathic disorder
A persistent disorder or disability of mind (whether or not including significant impairment of intelligence) which results in abnormally aggressive or seriously irresponsible conduct on the part of the person concerned.

Patient

A person having or appearing to have a mental disorder.

Medical treatment

Includes nursing and care and rehabilitation under medical supervision.

Responsible Medical Officer

The registered medical practitioner in charge of the treatment of the patient, i.e. the consultant psychiatrist; if he or she is not available the doctor who for the time being is in charge of the patient's treatment may deputize.

Approved Doctor

A registered medical practitioner approved under Section 12 of the Act by the Secretary of State (with authority being delegated to the Regional Health Authority) as having special experience in the diagnosis or treatment of mental disorder.

Approved Social Worker

An officer of a local social services authority with appropriate training who may make applications for compulsory admission; hospital senior social workers usually hold lists of Approved Social Workers.

Nearest relative

The first surviving person in the following list, with full blood relatives taking preference over half-blood relatives, and the elder of two relatives of the same description or level of kinship also taking preference:

a. Husband or wife
b. Son or daughter
c. Father or mother
d. Brother or sister
e. Grandparent
f. Grandchild
g. Uncle or aunt
h. Nephew or niece.

Preference is also given to a relative with whom the patient ordinarily lives or by whom he or she is cared for.

It should be noted that the Mental Health Act does not define the term 'mental illness'; its operational definition is a matter of clinical judgement in each individual case.

So far as the definition of 'mental disorder' is concerned, the Act states that a person may *not* be dealt with under the Mental Health Act as having a mental disorder 'by reason only of promiscuity or other immoral conduct, sexual deviancy or dependence on alcohol or drugs'.

SECTION 2: ADMISSION FOR ASSESSMENT

Purpose

To admit a patient to hospital for assessment.

Grounds

The patient has a mental disorder of a nature or degree that warrants his or her detention in a hospital for assessment (or for assessment followed by medical treatment) for at least a limited period; *and* the patient ought to be so detained in the interests of his or her own health or safety or with a view to protecting others.

Medical recommendations

By two medical practitioners:

- One medical practitioner must be an Approved Doctor.
- Other than in exceptional circumstances, the second medical recommendation should be provided by a doctor having previous knowledge of the patient. In the case of the general practitioner, 'having previous knowledge' includes general practitioners in the same practice who have discussed the patient. Where this is not possible, for example if the patient is not registered with a general practitioner, then it is desirable for the second medical recommendation to be provided by an Approved Doctor.

The two doctors should agree and state that the two grounds for making the recommendation are complied with. They should ideally examine the patient together, and then go on to complete and sign joint medical recommendation forms (forms 3) at the same time. If they examine the patient separately, not more than 5 clear days should have elapsed between the two examinations, and separate recommendation forms should be used (forms 4).

Applications

May be made by an Approved Social Worker or the nearest relative, either of whom must have seen the patient within 14 days, ending with the date of application. The Approved Social Worker is usually the right applicant, in view of his or her professional training, knowledge of the legislation and of local resources, together with the potential adverse effect that a nearest relative application might have on the relationship with the patient. The doctor should advise the nearest relative that it is preferable for an Approved Social Worker to make an assessment of the need for the patient to be compulsorily admitted, and for the Approved Social Worker to make the application if deemed necessary. The Code of Practice (1990) states that the doctor should never advise the nearest relative to make the application so as to avoid an Approved Social Worker in an assessment.

Duration

Up to 28 days, starting with the day of admission. The patient must be discharged at the end of this period unless further powers of detention have been taken.

Powers of discharge

The doctor in charge of the case, the hospital managers or the nearest relative may discharge the patient, but the managers may prevent the discharge by the nearest relative if the doctor in charge of the case certifies that the patient is dangerous. In this case the nearest relative may apply to a Tribunal within 28 days. The patient may apply to a Mental Health Review Tribunal within the first 14 days of detention.

Pointers to compulsory admission under Section 2

In deciding whether to use Section 2 or Section 3 (see below) the Code of Practice (1990) gives the following pointers to using Section 2 rather than Section 3:

- Where the diagnosis and prognosis of a patient's condition are unclear
- There is a need to carry out an inpatient assessment to formulate a treatment plan
- Where a judgement is needed as to whether a patient will accept treatment on a voluntary basis following admission

- Where a patient who has already been assessed, and who has been previously admitted compulsorily under the Mental Health Act, is judged to have changed since the previous admission and needs further assessment
- Where a patient has not previously been admitted either compulsorily or informally.

SECTION 3: ADMISSION FOR TREATMENT

Purpose
The compulsory admission of a patient for the treatment of his or her mental disorder.

Grounds
The patient has a mental illness, severe mental impairment, psychopathic disorder or mental impairment of a nature or degree that makes it appropriate for him or her to receive medical treatment in hospital; *and* in the case of psychopathic disorder or mental impairment such treatment is likely to alleviate or prevent a deterioration of his or her condition; *and* it is necessary for the health or safety of other persons that the patient should receive such treatment, which cannot be provided unless he or she is detained under Section 3.

Medical recommendations
By two medical practitioners, as in the case of Section 2. The joint medical recommendation forms used are forms 10; if the patient is seen separately by the two doctors, then separate recommendation forms (forms 11) are used.

Applications
As for Section 2. An objection from the nearest relative prevents the Approved Social Worker making the application for Section 3.

Duration
Up to 6 months. May then be renewed for a further 6 months by the Responsible Medical Officer, and then at annual intervals.

Powers of discharge
The patient may be discharged by the Responsible Medical Officer, by the hospital managers or by the nearest relative,

having given 72 hours notice, unless the Responsible Medical Officer has certified that the patient is dangerous. In this case the nearest relative may apply to a Mental Health Review Tribunal, on behalf of the patient, within 28 days of being so informed.

The patient may appeal to a Mental Health Review Tribunal within 6 months of admission. If this does not happen and the patient is detained for a further 6 months, the hospital managers must automatically refer the case to the Tribunal.

Pointers to compulsory admission under Section 3

In deciding whether to use Section 2 or Section 3 the Code of Practice (1990) gives the following pointers to using Section 3 rather than Section 2:

- Where a patient has been admitted in the past, is considered to need compulsory admission for the treatment of a mental disorder which is already known to the clinical team, and has been assessed in the recent past by that team
- Where a patient already admitted under Section 2 who is assessed as needing further medical treatment for mental disorder under the Mental Health Act at the conclusion of the detention under Section 2 is unwilling to remain in hospital informally and to consent to the medical treatment
- Where a patient is detained under Section 2 and assessment points to a need for treatment under the Mental Health Act for a period beyond the 28-day detention under Section 2. In such circumstances an application for detention under Section 3 should be made at the earliest opportunity and should not be delayed until the end of the Section 2 detention.

Section 2 should *not* be used instead of Section 3 to avoid consulting the nearest relative or because the proposed treatment to be administered under the Mental Health Act is likely to last less than 28 days.

SECTION 4: ADMISSION IN AN EMERGENCY

Purpose

Emergency application for admission for assessment.

Grounds

It is of urgent necessity for the patient to be admitted and detained in hospital under Section 4 of the Mental Health Act (and for the reasons given under Section 2).

Medical recommendations

May be limited to just one of the two medical practitioners required in the case of Section 2 (who does not have to be an Approved Doctor). The patient should be admitted within 24 hours of the medical examination (or of the application if earlier).

Applications

The nearest relative or an Approved Social Worker, either of whom must have seen the patient within the previous 24 hours.

Duration

Lasts 72 hours from the time of admission.

Powers of discharge

By the end of the 72 hours one of the following options is implemented:

- The patient is discharged
- The patient remains informally
- A second medical recommendation is received which, together with the first medical recommendation, allows the requirements for detention under Section 2 to be complied with
- Application for compulsory admission under Section 3 is initiated.

There are no appeal procedures.

••

AIMS

The general aims of Sections 2, 3 and 4 of the Mental Health Act are as follows:

- To allow compulsory admission of a patient with a mental disorder so that assessment and/or treatment can take place

- To protect others who may be at risk from the patient if he or she were not admitted
- To safeguard those who are not mentally disordered from being inappropriately detained compulsorily.

Appendix II: ICD-10 Classification

This appendix briefly outlines the tenth revision of the *International classification of diseases* (ICD-10), published by the World Health Organization in 1992.

Organic, including symptomatic, mental disorders

F00 Dementia in Alzheimer's disease
F01 Vascular dementia
F02 Dementia in other diseases classified elsewhere
F03 Unspecified dementia
F04 Organic amnesic syndrome, not induced by alcohol and other psychoactive substances
F05 Delirium, not induced by alcohol and other psychoactive substances
F06 Other mental disorders due to brain damage and dysfunction and to physical disease
F07 Personality and behavioural disorders due to brain disease, damge and dysfunction
F09 Unspecified organic or symptomatic mental disorder.

Mental and Behavioural disorders resulting from psychoactive substance use

F10 Mental and behavioural disorders due to use of alcohol
F11 Mental and behavioural disorders due to use of opioids
F12 Mental and behavioural disorders due to use of cannabinoids
F13 Mental and behavioural disorders due to use of sedatives or hypnotics
F14 Mental and behavioural disorders due to use of cocaine

F15   Mental and behavioural disorders due to use of other stimulants, including caffeine
F16   Mental and behavioural disorders due to use of hallucinogens
F17   Mental and behavioural disorders due to use of tobacco
F18   Mental and behavioural disorders due to use of volatile solvents
F19   Mental and behavioural disorders due to multiple drug use and use of other psychoactive substances.

Schizophrenia, schizotypal and delusional disorders

F20   Schizophrenia
F21   Schizotypal disorder
F22   Persistent delusional disorders
F23   Acute and transient psychotic disorders
F24   Induced delusional disorder
F25   Schizoaffective disorder
F28   Other non-organic psychotic disorders
F29   Unspecified non-organic psychosis

Mood (affective) disorders

F30   Manic episode
F31   Bipolar affective disorder
F32   Depressive episode
F33   Recurrent depressive disorder
F34   Persistent mood (affective) disorders
F35   Other mood (affective) disorders
F39   Unspecified mood (affective) disorder

Neurotic, stress-related and somatoform disorders

F40   Phobic anxiety disorders
F41   Other anxiety disorders
F42   Obsessive–compulsive disorder
F43   Reaction to severe stress, and adjustment disorders
F44   Dissociative (conversion) disorders
F45   Somatoform disorders
F48   Other neurotic disorders

Behavioural syndromes associated with physiological disturbances and physical factors

F50   Eating disorders
F51   Non-organic sleep disorders
F52   Sexual dysfunction, not caused by organic disorder or disease
F53   Mental and behavioural disorders associated with the puerperium, not elsewhere classified
F54   Psychological and behavioural factors associated with disorders or diseases classified elsewhere
F55   Abuse of non-dependence-producing substances
F59   Unspecified behavioural syndromes associated with physiological disturbances and physical factors

Disorders of adult personality and behaviour

F60   Specific personality disorders
F61   Mixed and other personality disorders
F62   Enduring personality changes, not attributable to brain damage and disease
F63   Habit and impulse disorders
F64   Gender identity disorders
F65   Disorders of sexual preference
F66   Psychological and behavioural disorders associated with sexual development and orientation
F68   Other disorders of adult personality and behaviour
F69   Unspecified disorder of adult personality and behaviour

Mental retardation

F70   Mild mental retardation
F71   Moderate mental retardation
F72   Severe mental retardation
F73   Profound mental retardation
F78   Other mental retardation
F79   Unspecified mental retardation

Disorders of psychological development

F80   Specific developmental disorders of speech and language

F81   Specific developmental disorders of scholastic skills
F82   Specific developmental disorders of motor function
F83   Mixed specific developmental disorders
F84   Pervasive developmental disorders
F88   Other disorders of psychological development
F89   Unspecified disorder of psychological development

Behavioural and emotional disorders with onset usually occurring in childhood and adolescence

F90   Hyperkinetic disorders
F91   Conduct disorders
F92   Mixed disorders of conduct and emotions
F93   Emotional disorders with onset specific to childhood
F94   Disorders of social functioning with onset specific to childhood and adolescence
F95   Tic disorders
F98   Other behavioural and emotional disorders with onset usually occurring in childhood and adolescence

Unspecified mental disorder

F99   Mental disorder, not otherwise specified

Appendix III: DSM-IV Classification

....

This appendix briefly outlines the fourth edition of the *Diagnostic and statistical manual of mental disorders* (DSM-IV), published by the American Psychiatric Association in 1994. It is a multiaxial classification with the following five axes:

Axis I Clinical disorders
        Other conditions that may be a focus of clinical attention
Axis II Personality disorders
         Mental retardation
Axis III General medical conditions
Axis IV Psychosocial and environmental problems
Axis V Global assessment of functioning.

In the following summary NOS stands for 'not otherwise specified'.

....

AXIS I: CLINICAL DISORDERS; OTHER CONDITIONS THAT MAY BE A FOCUS OF CLINICAL ATTENTION

Disorders usually first diagnosed in infancy, childhood or adolescence (excluding mental retardation, which is diagnosed on axis II)

Learning disorder
Motor skills disorder
Communication disorders
Pervasive developmental disorder
- Autistic disorder
- Rett's disorder
- Childhood disintegrative disorder
- Asperger's disorder
- NOS

Attention-deficit and disruptive behaviour disorders
Feeding and eating disorders of infancy and early childhood
Tic disorders
Elimination disorders
–   Encopresis
–   Enuresis
Other disorders of infancy, childhood or adolescence

Delirium, dementia and amnestic and other cognitive disorders
Delirium
Dementia
Amnestic disorders
Other cognitive disorders

Mental disorders resulting from a general medical condition
Substance-related disorders
Alcohol-related disorders
Amphetamine (or amphetamine-like)-related disorders
Caffeine-related disorders
Cannabis-related disorders
Cocaine-related disorders
Hallucinogen-related disorders
Inhalant-related disorders
Nicotine-related disorders
Opioid-related disorders
Phencyclidine (or phencyclidine-like)-related disorders
Sedative-, hypnotic- or anxiolytic-related disorders
Polysubstance-related disorders
Other (or unknown) substance-related disorders

Schizophrenia and other psychotic disorders
Schizophrenia
Schizophreniform disorder
Schizoaffective disorder
Delusional disorder
Brief psychotic disorder
Shared psychotic disorder
Psychotic disorder resulting from a general medical condition

Substance-induced psychotic disorder
Psychotic disorder NOS

Mood disorders
Depressive disorders
Bipolar disorders

Anxiety disorders
Panic disorder without agoraphobia
Panic disorder with agoraphobia
Agoraphobia without history of panic disorder
Specific phobia
Social phobia
Obsessive–compulsive disorder
Post-traumatic stress disorder
Acute stress disorder
Generalized anxiety disorder
Anxiety disorder resulting from a general medical condition
Substance-induced anxiety disorder
NOS

Somatoform disorder
Somatization disorder
Undifferentiated somatoform disorder
Conversion disorder
Pain disorder
Hypochondriasis
Body dysmorphic disorder
NOS

Factitious disorder
Dissociative disorder
Dissociative amnesia
Dissociative fugue
Dissociative identity disorder
Depersonalization disorder
NOS

Sexual and gender identity disorders
Sexual dysfunctions
– Sexual desire disorders
– Sexual arousal disorders

- Orgasmic disorders
- Sexual pain disorders
- Sexual dysfunction resulting from a general medical condition

Paraphilias
- Exhibitionism
- Fetishism
- Frotteurism
- Paedophilia
- Sexual masochism
- Sexual sadism
- Transvestic fetishism
- Voyeurism
- NOS

Gender identity disorders

Eating disorders
Anorexia nervosa
Bulimia nervosa
NOS

Sleep disorders
Primary sleep disorders
- Dyssomnias
- Parasomnias

Sleep disorders related to another medical disorder
Other sleep disorders

Impulse-control disorders not elsewhere classified

Adjustment disorders

Other conditions that may be a focus of clinical attention

AXIS II: PERSONALITY DISORDERS; MENTAL RETARDATION

Personality disorders
Paranoid personality disorder
Schizoid personality disorder
Schizotypal personality disorder
Antisocial personality disorder
Antisocial personality disorder

Borderline personality disorder
Histrionic personality disorder
Narcissistic personality disorder
Avoidant personality disorder
Dependent personality disorder
Obsessive–compulsive personality disorder
NOS

Mental retardation
Mild mental retardation
Severe mental retardation
Profound mental retardation
Mental retardation, severity unspecified

AXIS III: GENERAL MEDICAL CONDITIONS

Infectious and parasitic diseases
Neoplasms
Endocrine, nutritional and metabolic diseases, and immunity disorders
Diseases of the blood and blood-forming organs
Diseases of the nervous system and sense organs
Diseases of the circulatory system
Diseases of the respiratory system
Diseases of the digestive system
Diseases of the genitourinary system
Complications of pregnancy, childbirth and the puerperium
Diseases of the skin and subcutaneous tissue
Diseases of the musculoskeletal system and connective tissue
Congenital anomalies
Certain conditions originating in the perinatal period
Symptoms, signs and ill-defined conditions
Injury and poisoning

AXIS IV: PSYCHOSOCIAL AND ENVIRONMENTAL PROBLEMS

Problems with primary support group
Problems related to the social environment
Educational problems
Occupational problems

Housing problems
Economic problems
Problems with access to health care services
Problems related to interaction with the legal system/crime
Other psychosocial and environmental problems

AXIS V: GLOBAL ASSESSMENT OF FUNCTIONING

Axis V is for reporting the clinician's judgement of the individual's overall level of functioning. This information is useful in planning treatment and measuring its impact, and in predicting outcome.

Glossary

....

acute intoxication a transient condition following the administration of a psychoactive substance, causing changes in physiological, psychological or behavioural functions and responses

affect pattern of observable behaviours which is the expression of a subjectively experienced feeling state (emotion) and is variable over time in response to changing emotional states

agitation excessive motor activity with a feeling of inner tension

agnosic alexia words can be seen but not read

agoraphobia literally a fear of the marketplace. A generalized high anxiety level with multiple phobic symptoms. It may include a fear of crowds, open and closed spaces, and travelling by public transport

alexithymia difficulty in being aware of or describing one's emotions

ambitendency a series of tentative, incomplete movements carried out when a voluntary action is anticipated

ambivalence simultaneous presence of opposing impulses towards the same thing

amnesia inability to recall past experiences

amok seen in southeast Asia. Following a depressive episode there is an outburst of aggressive behaviour in which the patient runs amok

anhedonia inability to feel enjoyment

anosognosia lack of awareness of disease

anxiety feeling of apprehension or tension caused by anticipating an external or internal danger

apathy detachment or indifference, and a loss of emotional tone and the ability to feel pleasure

attention ability to focus on an activity

automatism act over which a person has no control, e.g. sleepwalking

autoscopy (phantom mirror image)   hallucination in which one sees and recognizes oneself

autopagnosia   inability to name, recognize or point on command to parts of the body

blunted affect   reduction in emotional expression

Capgras' syndrome   a person who is familiar to the patient is believed to have been replaced by a double

central (syntactical) aphasia   difficulty in arranging words in their correct sequence

circumstantiality   slowed thinking incorporating unnecessary trivial details. The goal of thought is finally, but slowly, reached

clanging   speech in which words are chosen because of their sounds rather than their meanings. It includes rhyming and punning

clouding of consciousness   the patient is drowsy and does not react completely to stimuli. There is disturbance of attention, concentration, memory, orientation and thinking

coenestopathic state   localized distortion of body awareness

coma   in deep coma there is no response to deep pain or any spontaneous movement. Tendon, pupillary and corneal reflexes are usually absent

compulsions or compulsive rituals   repetitive, stereotyped, seemingly purposeful behaviour which is the motor component of obsessional thoughts, e.g. checking and cleaning rituals

concentration   ability to sustain attention

concrete thinking   lack of abstract thinking, normal in childhood, and occurring in adults with organic brain disease and schizophrenia

confabulation   gaps in memory are unconsciously filled with false memories

Cotard's syndrome   nihilistic delusional disorder in which, for example, patients believes their money, friends or body parts do not exist

countertransference   therapist's emotions and attitudes to the patient

culture-bound syndromes   specific psychiatric disorders occurring in certain non-western countries

defence mechanisms   mental mechanisms that protect consciousness from the affects, ideas and desires of the unconscious

déjà vu illusion of recognition of a situation

déjà pensé illusion of recognition of new thought

delirium disorder of consciousness in which the patient is bewildered, disoriented and restless. There may be associated fear and hallucinations

delusions of infidelity (pathological jealousy, delusional jealousy, Othello's syndrome) delusional belief that one's spouse or lover is being unfaithful

delusion of reference behaviour of others, and objects and events, e.g. television broadcasts, believed to refer to oneself in particular. When similar thoughts are held with less than delusional intensity they are ideas of reference

delusion false personal belief based on incorrect inference about external reality and firmly sustained in spite of both what almost everyone else believes and what constitutes incontrovertible and obvious proof or evidence to the contrary. The belief is not one normally held by others of the same subculture

delusion (illusion) or doubles (*I'illusion de sosies***)** delusional belief that a person known to the patient has been replaced by a double; it is seen in Capgras' syndrome

delusional perception new and delusional significance is attached to a familiar real perception without any logical reason

dementia global organic impairment of intellectual functioning without impairment of consciousness

denial defence mechanism in which the subject acts as if consciously unaware of a wish of reality

dependence syndrome use of psychoactive substances has a higher priority than other behaviours which once had higher value. There is a desire, often strong and over powering, to take the substance(s) on a continuous or periodic basis

depersonalization feeling that one is altered or not real in some way

depression low or depressed mood that may be accompanied by anhedonia, in which the ability to enjoy regular and pleasurable activities is lost. In normal grief or mourning the sadness is appropriate to the loss

depressive retardation lesser form of psychomotor retardation which occurs in depression

derealization surroundings do not seem real

disorders (loosening) of association (formal thought disorder) language disorder seen in schizophrenia, e.g. 'knight's move' thinking and word salad

displacement defence mechanism in which thoughts and feelings about one person or object are transferred onto another

dissociative disorder disorder in which there is a disturbance in the normal integration of awareness of identity, consciousness, memory and control of bodily movements

distractibility attention is frequently drawn to irrelevant external stimuli

DSM-IV fourth edition of the *Diagnostic and statistical manual of mental disorders*, published by the American Psychiatric Association, Washington DC (1994). It is a multiaxial classification with five axes

dysarthria difficulty articulating speech

dysphoria unpleasant mood

echolalia automatic imitation of another's speech

echopraxia automatic imitation of another's movements even when asked not to

ecstasy feeling of intense rapture

ego part of the mental apparatus that is present at the interface of the perceptual and internal demand systems. It controls voluntary thoughts and actions and, at an unconscious level, defence mechanisms

egomania pathological preoccupation with oneself

eidetic image vivid and detailed reproduction of a previous perception, e.g. a photographic memory

elevated mood mood more cheerful than normal. It is not necessarily pathological

erotomania (de Clérambault's syndrome) patient holds the delusional belief that someone else, usually of a higher social or professional status, is in love with them

euphoric mood exaggerated feeling of wellbeing. It is pathological

expansive mood feelings are expressed without restraint, and one's self-importance may be overrated

expressive (motor) aphasia difficulty in expressing thoughts in words while comprehension remains

extracampine hallucination hallucination occuring outside one's sensory field

fear anxiety caused by a recognized real danger

flat affect almost no emotional expression at all; the patient typically has an immobile face and monotonous voice

flight of ideas speech consists of a stream of accelerated thoughts with abrupt changes from topic to topic and no central direction. The connections between the thoughts may be based on chance relationships, verbal associations (e.g. alliteration and assonance), clang associations and distracting stimuli

formication somatic hallucination in which insects are felt to be crawling under one's skin

free association articulation, without censorship, of all thoughts that come to mind

free-floating anxiety pervasive and unfocused anxiety

Fregoli's syndrome patient believes that a familiar person, who is often believed to be the patient's persecutor, has taken on a different appearance

freudian slips (parapraxes) unconscious thoughts slipping through when censorship is off guard

fugue state of wandering from usual surroundings and loss of memory

functional hallucination stimulus causing the hallucination is experienced in addition to the hallucination

global aphasia both receptive and expressive aphasia present at the same time

hallucination false sensory perception in the absence of a real external stimulus. It is perceived as being located in objective space and as having the same realistic qualities as normal perceptions. It is not subject to conscious manipulation and only indicates a psychotic disturbance when there is also impaired reality testing

hallucinosis hallucinations (usually auditory) occuring in clear consciousness, e.g. in alcoholism

hemisomatognosis (hemidepersonalization) a limb is felt to be missing

hyperacusis increased sensitivity to sounds

hyperaethesia sensory distortion in which sensations appear increased

hyperkinesis overactivity, distractibility, excitability and impulsivity, e.g. in children

hypnagogic hallucination hallucination occurring while falling asleep. It occurs in normal people

hypnapompic hallucination hallucination occurring while waking from sleep. It occurs in normal people

hypoaesthesia sensory distortion in which sensations appear decreased

hypochondriasis preoccupation, not based on real organic pathology, with a fear of having a serious physical illness. Physical senstions are unrealistically interpreted as being abnormal

ICD-10 tenth revision of the *International classification of diseases* published by the World Health Organization, Geneva (1992)

id unconscious part of the mental apparatus which is partly made up of inherited instincts and partly by acquired, but repressed, components

ideas of reference *see under* delusion of reference

illusion false perception of a real external stimulus

inappropriate affect affect that is inappropriate to the circumstances, for example appearing cheerful immediately following the death of a loved one

induced psychosis *(folie à deux)* delusional disorder shared by two (or more) people who are closely related emotionally. One has a genuine psychotic disorder and his or her delusional system is induced in the other, who may be dependent or less intelligent

introjection and identification defence mechanisms by which the attitudes and behaviour of another are transposed into oneself, helping one cope with separation from that person

isolation defence mechanism in which certain thoughts are isolated from others

jamais vu illusion of failure to recognize a familiar situation

jargon aphasia incoherent, meaningless, neologistic speech occurs

Klüver–Bucy syndrome syndrome characterized by placidity, hyperorality, hypersexuality, hyper-metamorphosis and hyperphagia, resulting from bilateral destruction of the amygdaloid bodies of the limbic system

knight's move thinking odd, tangential associations between ideas, leading to disruptions in the smooth continuity of speech

labile affect affect repeatedly and rapidly shifts, for example from sadness to anger

learning disability (mental retardation) classified by DSM-IV and ICD-10 as an intelligence quotient of less than 70

logoclonia last syllable of the last word is repeated

logorrhoea (volubility) fluent and rambling speech using many words

macropsia objects appear larger or nearer

made actions (made acts) delusional belief that one's free will has been removed and an external agency is controlling one's actions

made feelings delusional belief that one's free will has been removed and an external agency is controlling one's feelings

made impulses delusional belief that one's free will has been removed and an external agency is controlling one's impulses

mannerisms repeated, involuntary movements that appear to be goal directed

mens rea guilty state of mind at the time of a criminal offence

mental apparatus id, ego and superego in psychodynamic theory

micropsia objects appear smaller or farther away

mild mental retardation IQ of 50–70

moderate mental retardation IQ of 35–49

monomania pathological preoccupation with a single object

mood pervasive and sustained emotion which, in the extreme, markedly colours the person's perception of the world

mood-congruent delusion content of the delusion is appropriate to the patient's mood

mood-incongruent delusion content of the delusion is not inappropriate to the patient's mood

mutism total loss of speech

negativism motiveless resistance to commands and attempts to be moved

neologism word newly made up, or an everyday word used in a special way

neurosis neurotic disorder, that is, a psychiatric disorder in which the patient has insight into the illness, has only part of his or her personality involved in the disorder, can distinguish between subjective experiences and reality, and does not construct a false environment based on misconceptions

nihilistic delusion delusional belief that others, oneself or the world do not exist or are about to cease to exist

nominal aphasia difficulty in naming objects

obsessions repetitive, senseless thoughts recognized as being irrational by the patient which, at least initially, are unsuccessfully resisted

overvalued idea unreasonable and sustained intense preoccupation maintained with less than delusional intensity. The belief is demonstrably false and not one normally held by others of the same subculture. There is a marked associated emotional investment

palilalia word is repeated with increasing frequency

panic attacks acute, episodic, intense anxiety attacks with or without physiological symptoms

paraeidolia vivid imagery occurring without conscious effort while looking at a poorly structured background

paramnesia distorted recall leading to falsification of memory, e.g. confabulation, *déjà vu*, *déjà pensé*, *jamais vu*, retrospective falsification

passing by the point (vorbeigehen) answers to questions, though obviously wrong, show that the questions have been understood, e.g. asked 'What colour is grass?', the patient may answer 'Blue'. It is seen in Ganser's syndrome, first described in criminals awaiting trial

passivity phenomena delusional belief that an external agency is controlling aspects of the self which are normally entirely under one's own control (e.g. thought alienation, made feelings, made impulses, made actions, somatic passivity)

perseveration (of speech and movement) mental operations carry on beyond the point at which they are appropriate

personality disorders deeply ingrained and enduring behaviour patterns manifesting as inflexible responses to a broad range of personal and social situations

phantom limb following the removal of a limb there is a continued awareness of its presence

phobia persistent irrational fear of an activity, object or situation leading to avoidance. The fear is out of proportion to the real danger and cannot be reasoned away, being out of voluntary control

phobic anxiety focus of anxiety is avoided

physical dependence adaptive state in which intense physical disturbance occurs when the administration of a psychoactive substance is suspended. There is a desire to take the substance to avoid the physical symptoms of the withdrawal state

posturing an inappropriate or bizarre bodily posture adopted continuously over a long period

poverty of speech very reduced speech, sometimes with monosyllabic answers to questions

pressure of speech increased quantity and rate of speech which is difficult to interrupt

primary delusion delusion arising fully formed without any discernible connection with previous events. It may be preceded by a delusional mood, in which there is an awareness of something unusual and threatening occurring

profound mental retardation IQ of less than 20

projection defence mechanism in which repressed thoughts and wishes are attributed to other people or objects

projective identification defence mechanism in which another person is both seen as possessing and constrained to take on repressed aspects of oneself

prosopagnosia inability to recognize faces

pseudodementia similar clinically to dementia but has a non-organic cause, e.g. depression

pseudohallucination form of imagery arising in the subjective inner space of the mind and lacking the substantiality of normal perceptions. It is not subject to conscious manipulation

psychological dependence psychoactive substance producing a feeling of satisfaction and a psychological drive which requires periodic or continuous administration of the substance to produce pleasure or to avoid the psychological discomfort of its absence

psychomotor agitation excess (usually unproductive) overactivity and restlessness, e.g. in agitated depression

psychosis psychotic disorder in which the patient does not have insight, has the whole of his or her personality distorted by illness, and constructs a false environment out of subjective experiences. Delusions and/or hallucinations may occur

pure word deafness words that are heard cannot be comprehended

rationalization defence mechanism in which an attempt is made to explain in a logically consistent or ethically acceptable way affects, ideas and wishes the true motive of which is not consciously perceived

reaction formation defence mechanism in which a psychological attitude diametrically opposed to an oppressed wish is held

receptive (sensory) aphasia difficulty in comprehending word meanings

reduplication phenomenon part or all the body is felt to be duplicated

reflex hallucination stimulus in one sensory field leads to a hallucination in another

regression defence mechanism in which there is a return to an earlier stage of development

repression defence mechanism in which there is a pushing away of unacceptable affects, ideas and wishes so that they remain in the unconscious

retrospective falsification false details are added to the recollection of an otherwise real memory

selective inattention anxiety-provoking stimuli are blocked out

semicoma a semicomatose patient withdraws from the source of pain but does not show spontaneous motor activity

severe mental retardation IQ of 20–34

simple phobia fear of discrete objects (e.g. spiders) or situations

simultanagnosia a type of visual agnosia in which there is an inability globally to appreciate pictures, with preserved perception of detail

social phobia fear of personal interactions in a public setting, e.g. public speaking and eating in public

somatic passivity delusional belief that one is a passive recipient of bodily sensations from an external agency

somnambulism sleepwalking

somnolence patient who is drowsy or somnolent can be awoken by mild stimuli and can speak comprehensibly, perhaps for only a short while before falling asleep again

stammering flow of speech is broken by pauses and the repetition of parts of words

stereotypy repeated, regular fixed pattern of movement or speech that is not goal-directed

sublimation defence mechanism allowing unconscious wishes to be satisfied by means of socially acceptable activities

superego derivative of the ego which exercises self-judgement and holds ethical and moralistic values

synaesthesia stimulus in one sensory field leading to hallucination in another

systematized delusion group of delusions united by a single theme or a delusion with multiple elaborations

tactile (haptic) hallucinations superficial somatic hallucinations

talking past the point (vorbeireden) the point of what is being said is never quite reached

tension unpleasant increase in psychomotor activity

thought alienation delusional belief that one's thoughts are under the control of an outside agency or that others are participating in one's thinking. It includes thought insertion, thought withdrawal and thought broadcasting

thought blocking sudden interruption in the train of thought occurs, leaving a 'blank', after which what was being said cannot be recalled

thought broadcasting delusional belief that one's thoughts are being 'read' by others, as if they were being broadcast

thought insertion delusional belief that thoughts are being put into one's mind by an external agency

thought withdrawal delusional belief that thoughts are being removed from one's mind by an external agency

tics repeated, irregular movements involving a muscle group

tolerance the desired central nervous system effects of a psychoactive substance diminish with repeated use, so that increasing doses are needed to achieve the same effects

trailing phenomenon moving objects are seen as a series of discrete discontinuous images. It is associated with hallucinogens

transference unconscious process in which emotions and attitudes experienced in childhood are transferred to the therapist

undoing (what has been done) defence mechanism in which previous thoughts or actions are made not to have occurred

visceral hallucinations somatic hallucinations of deep sensations

visual asymbolia words can be transcribed but not read

waxy flexibility (cerea flexibilitas) the examiner, as he or she moves part of the patient's body, has a feeling of plastic resistance as if bending of a soft wax rod. The bodily part remains 'moulded' in its new position

withdrawal state physical and psychological symptoms, which may be complicated by delirium or convulsions, occur following absolute or relative withdrawal of a psychoactive substance after its repeated use

word salad (schizophasia or speech confusion) the speech is an incoherent and incomprehensible mix of words and phrases

Index